The Good Nutrients Guide

■The Good Nutrients Guide

The complete handbook of vitamins, minerals and other nutrients

Rita Greer and Robert Woodward

J. M. Dent & Sons Ltd
London   Melbourne

First published 1985
Copyright © Rita Greer and Robert Woodward 1985

Set in 9½ on 10½ pt Trump Medieval Roman by
The Word Factory, Rossendale, Lancs.
Printed in Great Britain by
Mackays of Chatham Ltd, for
J. M. Dent & Sons Ltd
33 Welbeck Street, London W1M 8LX

British Library Cataloguing in Publication Data

Greer, Rita
    The good nutrients guide.
    1. Nutrition
    I. Title   II. Woodward, Robert
    613.2   TX353

    ISBN 0–460–02298–9

■Contents

■Introduction

There are many other specialized books available on nutrition and the food elements essential for life, but this one is designed to cover the nutrients which will be found particularly (and sometimes exclusively) in fresh foods as well as in the bottles of products found in health stores, dietetic stores, pharmacies and vitamin bars in the developed world.

Understanding the mass of information which is now available to us on the subject of vital nutrients is a hard task for anyone unless the explanations are simple. The authors hope to give a fair, all-round picture of present-day knowledge by presenting not just the proven scientific facts already discovered but popular beliefs and myths, perhaps folklore, as well as hopes for future research. They will also show how vitamins and other nutrients are manufactured, advertised and controlled. This has involved an honest approach which we hope will be more welcome than wild claims and half truths that seem to abound on the subject and that do wonders for the sales of supplements in pill form.

What we call meals are really mixtures of food and within them will be found the so-called micronutrients which you probably know better as vitamins, minerals and trace elements. Many of the micronutrients are considered to be highly controversial from a scientific point of view, like all new advances in science. (It is only when such advances become accepted that they stop being controversial.) It is unlikely that all such items will eventually be accepted but we have included them in this book as part of our policy to present a broad outlook on the subject.

The basic idea that the kind of food we eat may help prevent disease and illness concerns a type of preventive health care which is called 'holistic'. In this approach not just single symptoms are treated but rather the whole person. This philosophy must not be confused with the view of established medical thinking – that there is a wonder drug or single chemical substance which will somehow prevent every symptom. Single vitamins or nutrients

1

are never enough on their own. They must be used with an overall nutritional treatment regime. Very often there is no need to take 'pills', and an adjustment in diet to ensure greater quantities of particular nutrients is all that is needed to combat a health problem. You will find recipes and dietary advice to help in this respect.

Supplementing the diet with 'vitamin pills' is considered by some nutritionists to be an outrageous idea and quite unnecessary. Medical practitioners who believe in holistic and preventive medicine take the opposite view and believe such supplements are an essential part of treatments. The whole question of diet supplementation is still controversial and will probably remain so for some time. The authors both believe supplements can have a role to play in nutrition if used sensibly but that they should only be used if reorganization of the diet fails to produce the extra nutrients needed. In other words, get your food right first before you start taking supplements.

Methods of manufacture and the many varieties of finished products available on the market are discussed with their respective merits or disadvantages. The authors hope this will be useful information for people who want to buy supplements and who are perplexed and confused by the vast array of bottles and packets in health food stores and pharmacies.

Probably the most fascinating research into nutrients this century has been the work done on vitamins and minerals, yet it is a comparatively neglected area of science. We hope this book will help to inform and also be of practical use in understanding and promoting micronutrients in preventive health care.

■1 Short history of nutrients

From earliest times one particular influence of food in relation to disease has been recognized. This is the knowledge that the decay of food leads to contamination and it is a major factor in the religious food laws of many kinds of belief, such as those of the Jewish faith.

In some sects milk and meat are not eaten at the same meal. As both of these quickly 'go off' in hot climates, by eating only one at a meal the risk of becoming ill afterwards is reduced by half. Pork is not eaten at all as it is a meat that does not keep well even in a cold climate and it is prone to parasitic infection. The kosher method of preparing meat after it has been killed is to salt it. Not only does this help to preserve but it removes most of the blood – the first part of the meat to go bad.

Such strict dietary laws, when first made, were based on commonsense and experience. Food that goes bad is easily identified by how it looks and smells. The link between eating food which has gone bad and its effects on people is usually very obvious. Scientific research, many centuries later, has proved how sensible most of the laws were in relation to poor standards of food hygiene. From a practical point of view the religious food laws have worked perfectly well for centuries, with or without scientific backing.

Today we know a great deal about bacteria and poisonous contaminants, thanks to modern science. We also know about diseases caused by nutrient deficiencies brought about by poor diet. There are historical references to such diseases as pellagra, rickets, beriberi and scurvy from as long ago as the second century BC. Intuition, inspired guesswork, commonsense or mere imagination were sometimes the tools of the early doctors and scientists whereas now we have organic chemistry and many branches of science, laboratories filled with the most amazing equipment and even computers to help unravel nutritional mysteries. This does not mean to say the early doctors and scientists were not right about some things, for they often were, but they did not know *why* they were right.

Not knowing why resulted in two things. Firstly, progress was slowed right down, often to a standstill; and secondly, their discoveries were not generally taken seriously and so were of little value.

A good example to illustrate these points is that of the disease scurvy which has an interesting history. Symptoms include bleeding gums, loose teeth, non-healing of wounds and almost unbearable joint pains. It was prevalent among sailors for centuries when sea voyages undertaken in sailing ships, before the days of steam or more sophisticated power, meant long periods at sea often with poor food – usually dry biscuits, dried meat and small beer. Some provisions were bought on route when the ships docked at various ports, if they were available or could be afforded. Fresh foods were avoided as they quickly deteriorated.

By today's standards the diet was extremely poor and obviously lacking in the fruit and vegetables which we now know are necessary for vital nutrients (vitamins and minerals). Voyages took months or years in some cases and crews often suffered badly from the mysterious disease.

As long ago as 1601 the East India Company discovered it could remove the risk of scurvy from its ships by giving the crews fresh lemon juice. No one knew how it worked but it was extremely successful. However, not every shipping line or navy followed suit and scurvy continued to be a scourge for many sailors. Later, in the eighteenth century, several researchers confirmed the earlier experiences of the East India Company – John Woodall (1639), Kramer (1793) and Lind (1753). In 1734 Bachstrom showed that sprouted seeds and grain could also be used to treat the disease. Sensible Captain Cook always took on supplies of fresh fruit for his crews when his ships called at ports, and scurvy was unknown among his sailors.

In spite of these examples of controlling scurvy, when it broke out in Ireland during the Potato Famine (1845–1847) no one knew quite what to do. It continued and in the nineteenth century it plagued sailors whose diets still provided too little in the way of vegetables and fruit. It finally took until the twentieth century for real progress in finding out the cause of the disease.

One factor which helped to speed up the work considerably was the important discovery that some animals, as well as humans, can also suffer from scurvy. By experimenting with the diet of guinea pigs, scientists were able to isolate a particular nutrient and then prove that scurvy is actually caused by *lack of vitamin C*.

This breathtakingly simple answer to the problem still does not prevent cases of scurvy even today. Old people or those on low incomes, infants and those who have a poor diet are the most likely ones to show symptoms of the disease. Having the knowledge of the cause alone is not enough. *We also need to be able to put the knowledge to good use.*

It was not until the latter part of the nineteenth century that scientific research began to show that there was a definite link between curing certain diseases and the eating of particular foods. Before this there could only be guesswork. However, it took until 1912 to clarify the situation. A researcher called Hopkins published his own findings which confirmed earlier work by other scientists begun in Europe in the previous century. Hopkins called the substances he had found in food, which he believed essential for life and which could cure some diseases, 'accessory factors'. This term did not exactly capture the imagination but another researcher (called Funk) christened them 'vitamines' and this did appeal to people. We still use the term, although without the 'e', as 'vitamins'.

After Hopkins' work was published and accepted in scientific circles, came an avalanche of research into nutrients. As more 'vitamins' were discovered they were allotted letters of the alphabet. Some proved to be more complicated and required further divisions with numbers as well as a letter of the alphabet. Names were given to some already numbered vitamins. While some vitamins, it was found, were destroyed by heat, others were not. Some kinds of food are high in a particular vitamin while others contain none at all. Some can be extracted from foods, while others can even be manufactured artificially (synthesized).

What emerged was new knowledge of a whole group of micronutrients with quite different and varied jobs to do in the body, found in all kinds of foods. And with still more knowledge to come from future research, as yet new and undreamed of nutrients and the somewhat muddled state of existing knowledge, will science help us to use what it has discovered or will it lead us astray?

Our basic nutritional problem seems to have changed over the last few decades. Where we were once undernourished we are now overnourished. What will be the long-term effects of this? Why do people take so little interest in what food they eat? Why are manufacturers so uninterested in the nutritional value of the foods they produce? Why aren't governments more interested in nutrition?

Those of us who are involved in such controversies about the nutritional quality of the food we eat and its long-term effects on health have cause for concern. Scientific dogma backed by large vested interests, both for controlling and financing food and drugs manufacture, make formidable adversaries. Yet there are signs of a greater wisdom prevailing which is growing all the time. In the field of nutrition and its related role in health care, new ideas are flourishing. This has led to wide public interest in vitamins and other nutrients. Even doctors and scientists, the most sceptical breed of people, are now taking preventive medicine very seriously. There are encouraging indications that nutrition will soon begin to feature as more than just a minor subject in medical teaching. When it does become important we shall be on a par with the Ancient Greeks regarding this particular approach.

■2   Nutrition

□ What does nutrition mean?

The human body is an amazingly complex and wonderful 'machine', but it cannot function without a supply of *food*. The nutrients in food are needed for energy, movement, heat, growth, repair, general maintenance and sometimes reproduction. The body needs to be able to *digest* the food it takes in so that it can be used in various ways. Some foods have to be processed into more basic kinds of food or treated chemically within the body. Others do not require such elaborate processing and some pass through the body almost unchanged.

There are six basic types of nutrients and two basic non-nutrients found in food. The six nutrients are carbohydrate, fat, protein, vitamins, minerals, trace elements; the two non-nutrients are fibre and water.

Carbohydrates are needed to provide energy and help keep the body warm. By processing carbohydrate the body can produce heat and so be able to work and move. Excess carbohydrate can be made (by the body) into fat and stored for future use.

Fats are another source of energy for the body, even more concentrated than carbohydrate. Again, excess of this nutrient can be stored as body fat for future use as an energy provider.

Proteins are needed for repairing damage and growth. The body is able to convert excess protein into energy and heat as it does with carbohydrate.

Vitamins, minerals and trace elements are necessary for the efficient working of the body. As you will see later in this book, there are many of them and they have special jobs to do in the body.

Water and fibre, as we have already stated, although not classed as nutrients, are nevertheless very important. Water is absolutely essential for life and while the body can survive for a limited time without food, it must have water or it cannot function. Fibre is not considered to be essential, but without it life for the human body can be extremely uncomfortable.

Generally speaking most foods contain several nutrients, in varying amounts. Carrots, for instance, contain a little protein, a trace of fat, some carbohydrate, a good deal of water, a little sugar, fibre, and a selection of vitamins and minerals such as potassium, sodium, calcium, iron, zinc, vitamins B6, C and E, folic acid, biotin and pantothenic acid etc.

The basic categories of foods being meat, fish, eggs, milk and dairy products, cereals (grains), fats/oils, vegetables, fruit, nuts, sugars and beverages, a shopping basket containing several days' supply of food is likely to contain some of each category. This will provide what is called a 'mixed diet', taken into the body in the form of meals, snacks and single foods.

To keep healthy and well needs a supply of food that will yield the appropriate amounts and types of nutrients to cope with the kind of lifestyle the individual enjoys. Although the body is usually very adaptable to varying amounts and types of food, with no two days' food being exactly the same, eating too little will lead to malnutrition and, in severe cases, even starvation and death. The body wastes away as it cannot repair any damage, produce new growth or any energy.

Although the word 'malnutrition' is associated with eating too little, eating too much is also covered by the term. The result of continual overeating is usually obesity – gross overweight. By not taking in enough of some kinds of food, deficiency diseases can occur. For example, anaemia may be the result of not taking in enough iron-containing foods and scurvy can be the result of too little vitamin C in the diet. In some cases, although the body takes in ample nutrients in a wide variety of foods, it is unable to use them on account of some kind of physical damage to the digestive tract or some inability to function. Coeliacs, for instance, cannot digest some grain proteins. If they do eat them, damage can result in the small intestine. The damage prevents them from absorbing fats and can lead to undernutrition and poor health.

□*Digestion and absorption of nutrients*

The food that we eat needs to be processed by the body so that it can eventually pass into the bloodstream and then on into the body's cells. The act of processing, which varies according to each kind of food, is called 'digestion'. Some nutrients are small enough to pass straight into the bloodstream but these are very few. (Salt, alcohol and glucose are three such nutrients.) Most of the other foods we eat need to be broken down chemically and to achieve this the body produces *enzymes* which help to speed up the digestion process.

Diagram showing digestive tract

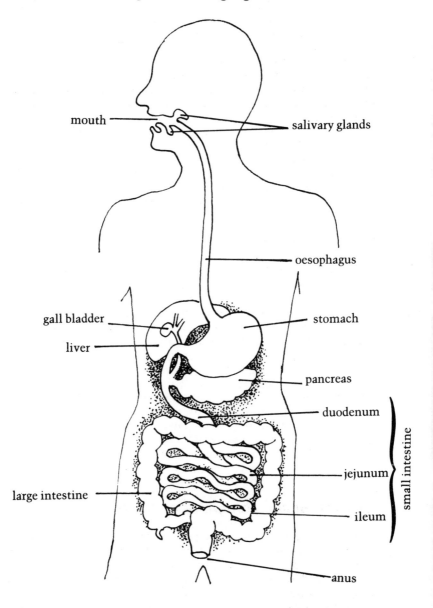

This diagram shows the various parts of the digestive tract discussed in the text that follows

Digestion takes place in the digestive tract. This comprises several complicated tubes all joined together to make one long tube about five metres long, starting with the mouth and ending with the anus. Surrounding the tube are body tissues which depend on the processed nutrients that the tube is able to produce from the food eaten. The lining of the tube varies and is constructed in such a way that the processed and chemically broken down nutrients can pass right through it and into the blood which can then carry them to where they are needed in the body.

The mouth is where the basic food supply enters the body, in quantity and often in quite large pieces. It is the job of the teeth to grind up the food into much smaller pieces. Three pairs of glands produce *saliva*. This helps to lubricate the pieces of food, making them easy to swallow and adding an enzyme whose job it is to begin work on breaking down the starch in food.

The part of the tube that joins the mouth to the stomach is called the oesophagus and after some processing in the mouth the food quickly passes down the oesophagus and collects in the stomach. The stomach enables us to eat meals (large amounts of food) instead of repeatedly eating small amounts of food, so it is in some respects a kind of food container. While food is in this container it is treated with three more enzymes which start work on processing the protein and fat in the food. Small quantities of water, alcohol, sugars, water-soluble minerals and some water-soluble vitamins can pass through the stomach wall into the bloodstream. However, most of the absorption takes place further on down the tube.

As well as the enzyme activity the stomach is also able to produce an acid that can destroy bacteria. This is hydrochloric acid and as well as being an antiseptic it works closely with one of the enzymes to speed up the digestion of protein. (It is only when there is an excessive amount of bacteria present that the acid fails to cope and infection or illness occurs.)

Because the acid is so powerful the stomach must really protect itself. It does this by producing a lining of mucus, a slimy substance. As if all this activity were not enough, the stomach is also capable of waves of muscular activity which can move the food about and so aid digestion. Foods rich in fat stay in the stomach longer than the ones with a high carbohydrate content. Depending on the type eaten, food will stay in the stomach from two to four hours, with the emotional state of the person also affecting the length of time it stays there.

After a thorough mixing, during which some enzyme activity takes place, the resulting mixture (chyme) is gradually forced out into the next part of the tube. This is called the small intestine, although it is actually as long as three metres and comprises three tubes joined together – the duodenum, the jejunum and the ileum.

As the activity in the stomach is such an acid affair, the small intestine enzyme juices make the food being processed slightly alkaline to neutralize the acid. Several enzymes are needed, especially those produced by the pancreas. This lies in the loop made by the first part of the small intestine (the duodenum). (You may have seen animal pancreas at the butcher's or supermarket, where it is sold as 'sweetbreads'.)

To help with the work of digesting carbohydrate and protein in the duodenum and also the absorption of vitamins A, D and K (all fat-soluble), the liver produces bile which enters through a duct into the duodenum. Bile is made continuously by the liver and stored in the gall bladder. Bile has another job to do as well. It plays a part in signalling the start of the digestive process, causing the saliva and gastric juices to begin flowing. This is not the only way digestive activity can start as there can be an element of mental stimulation too. (Close your eyes and imagine a lemon being cut in half. You should feel an increase in the flow of saliva in your mouth.) The muscular contractions of the duodenum set off the flow of bile into it from the gall bladder. This in turn stimulates the production of a hormone which encourages the pancreas to release enzymes to aid digestion in the small intestine. Bile contains bile salts which help in the digestion of fats by making them into minute droplets.

Most of the absorption of nutrients into the bloodstream takes place in the small intestine. This has an amazingly large surface area of about forty square metres because it is lined with hair-like structures (villi) which are themselves covered with even smaller 'hairs' (the brush border). They are needed to absorb water, alcohol, sugars, minerals, water soluble vitamins, broken-down proteins (amino acids), fatty acids, fat-soluble vitamins and broken-down starches.

The next part of the tube is called the large intestine and here the final stage in digestion takes place of any remaining food which has been processed but not yet absorbed. Most of the water in the food is also absorbed, leaving comparatively dry waste material and debris to be passed out of the body. The large intestine also provides the right conditions for helpful bacteria to grow. These will try to process any undigested food still left in the tube and in doing so can actually manufacture vitamins too, especially those of the B group.

Water can be absorbed through the stomach and both the small and large intestines. Excess water taken in by the body can usually be excreted via the kidneys in urine.

If the digestive tract is unable to process food fully enough for absorption to take place, that food becomes 'indigestible'. This can lead to problems as the body is unable to cope with the food in the normal way. Discomfort, flatulence (wind) and heartburn may be experienced. In more severe cases the result may be diarrhoea and pain. Emotional upsets can also cause indigestion.

□*Digestion in infants*

Digestion in infants is not the same as in adults. Before they are born, babies receive nutrients from the mother via the placenta into the bloodstream. For several weeks after birth no solid food can be taken and liquid food only is given to the baby, mainly in the form of milk. To cope with this the stomach contains a special enzyme (rennin) which can clot the casein in the milk and so enable its digestion to begin. The stomach of a baby is not equipped to digest starch until, after several months, the digestive tract has gradually developed into one comparable with that of an adult, able to take a mixture of foods including starches.

The fashion for very early weaning and introduction of solid foods far too soon has led to digestive problems for many babies. The popularity of bottle feeding with cow's milk instead of human milk can also cause problems in babies, although the pro cow's milk lobby do not accept this idea. (See page 39 for informative chart.)

As this book sets out to give information in simple terms, this explanation of digestion and absorption may seem oversimplified. Extra information follows concerning enzymes and other items not dealt with so far.

□*Extra facts about digestion and absorption*

Saliva This is secreted from glands at the back of the mouth and under the tongue. It is usually present in the mouth, which is therefore always ready to take in food. The sight, taste and smell of appetizing food can cause an increase in the flow of saliva from the glands. The enzyme ptyalin can help to convert some of the starch in food to maltose.

Gastric juice This is produced by the lining of the stomach and contains pepsin, an enzyme which starts to break down protein into peptides. In infants (only), the enzyme rennin acts on milk protein to turn it into peptides. (In the small intestine the peptides are split into amino acids and then absorbed into the bloodstream.)

Pancreatic enzymes

Three important enzymes are produced by the pancreas.

Trypsin is a very powerful enzyme that can quickly break down proteins, especially those in meat.

Amylase can break down starch. Very little amylase is made by the pancreas in an infant and this is why babies cannot easily digest starches.

Lipase is capable of splitting fats into fatty acids.

Small intestine enzymes

Peptidases can complete the breakdown of proteins.

Maltase, sucrase and lactase are supplementary enzymes that can split carbohydrates.

Intestinal lipase acts on fat in much the same way the pancreatic enzyme lipase does.

Bile A bilious attack, or in more severe form an attack of jaundice or obstruction of the tube connecting the liver with the gall bladder (bile duct), can cause an accumulation of bile in the blood. This can result in yellowing of the skin and whites of the eyes because of the yellow/green or reddish brown colour of the bile.

□*Basic nutrients and non-nutrients in the diet*

While a minority of people are born with an illness or disease, most illnesses are the result of something in our environment – extremes of temperature, the quality of the air we breathe, accident or civil unrest, war, terrorist attacks, 'acts of God', bacteria, infection, parasites, viruses, radiation, microwaves, and, most important in relation to this book, what we eat and drink.

Our protection against disease and injury can take many forms, for our bodies are well equipped to cope if they are in a healthy state – physical reactions to danger, instinctive reactions, protective antibody reactions, our complicated immune system, senses of taste, smell, sight and hearing. Not only do these mean we can survive in a hostile environment but they also help us to be healthy.

Because we live in heated buildings and not out in the open, we are unlikely to suffer from exposure. We also have sanitation, supplies of fresh water, drainage, soap and detergents to help us make the idea of hygiene a practical reality. We don't have fur or feathers to keep us warm, so we wear clothes. Our feet (especially the soles) are protected by shoes, and hats and gloves protect our head and hands when required. Inventions help our senses when they fail us – hearing aids, spectacles and sunglasses. Extra warm clothes can be worn in very cold climates and special creams can filter harmful rays of the sun on our skin.

The food and drink we consume is very varied. We import foods from other countries that we cannot produce ourselves so that we do not have to rely on just what can be produced in the latitude in which we live. For example, we can enjoy tropical fruits such as pineapples and bananas which could never be grown commercially in Britain.

Our diets usually contain all kinds of processed and fresh foods such as cereals (grains) and cereal products, cow's milk and products made from it, eggs, meat and meat products, fish, vegetables, fruit, nuts, sugars and beverages, fats and oils, and seeds. However, many people also take vitamin and mineral supplements as well as this varied diet.

Remember, the basic nutrients this kind of diet supplies are protein, fat, carbohydrate, fibre, water, vitamins, minerals and trace elements. Although water and fibre are not really nourishing, they are a very important part of the diet, as you will see.

Water

Two-thirds of our body weight is water and without a supply of it we die within a few days. (In many languages the word for water is the same as the word that means life.) Water and fibre together do a very important job within our bodies, probably best explained as 'cleansing and waste disposal'.

Fibre

The value of fibre in our diet has been very much overlooked in the past. This is because it has low levels of nutrients and until quite recently its valuable function in the body had not been fully understood or recognized. Very little research has been undertaken on fibre and there is very little information available on it in nutrition textbooks. However, the work by Cleave, Burkitt and Trowell this century on fibre in the diet of people in underdeveloped countries has made a positive contribution to our knowledge.

The word 'fibre' has become associated so closely with wheat bran that most people think that this is the only fibre available for us in our diet. However, the word has really a much wider meaning.

Fibre is nature's strong building and packaging material. It is found in quite large amounts in plants, in their stems, roots, leaves, pods and seeds. Consequently the best sources of fibre in our diet are cereals (grains), legumes, nuts and dried fruits. Fresh vegetables and fruit are lesser sources of fibre, contrary to popular belief.

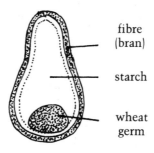

fibre (bran)

starch

wheat germ

To show you how fibre is used to package, here is a section through a wheat grain. Notice just how neatly it wraps up and strengthens the grain.

Celery is an example of how long fibres help to support the plant in its stalk formation. You can imagine just how weak it would be without these fibres. The stalks and veins on leafy plants such as cabbage contain more fibre than the green parts because they make the framework of the plant.

Although dietary fibre contains very little in the way of nourishment, it is nevertheless a very important part of our diet. A high intake of pectins may well reduce the risk of isachaemic heart disease by lowering the plasma cholesterol. Because of their bulkiness high fibre foods pass more slowly through the first part of the alimentary canal and this may reduce the risk of obesity and diabetes. Quicker movement of waste foods through the lower part of the canal may prove to mean less risk of cancer of the colon and rectum, and straining due to constipation, which is in turn due to slow transit times and may lead to hernia and haemorrhoids.

None of these facts is really proved yet to the satisfaction of modern science, except perhaps that a diet high in the right kind of fibre can prevent constipation. The hazards of a new diet phenomenon, the too-high-in-fibre-diet, are as yet unknown except that eating too much fibre, in some cases, can influence the amount of minerals we can absorb, especially zinc. Much more research is needed in this important field to prove just how valuable fibre may be as a protector of our health. We need to know much more about it to use it to our best advantage.

15

There are five main chemical types of dietary fibre provided by plants, trees, shrubs and seaweeds. (By chemical we mean in the language of chemistry, not that they are produced artificially.) These five types are cellulose and hemicellulose, lignins (which encrust cellulose and hemicellulose), pectins (found mainly in fruit), gums (from trees and shrubs) and mucilages (from seeds and seaweeds). These are all natural fibres.

Types of fibre

Wheat bran – used in breakfast cereals and for baking as a fibre boost.

Pea bran – used to increase the fibre content of some commercial breads, especially white loaves labelled 'with bran'.

Rice bran – made from rice husks and used for special diet food, especially food for wheat and gluten allergics.

Seed bran – also used for allergics as an alternative to wheat bran, e.g. husks of evening primrose seeds.

Soya bran – made from soya beans and used as an alternative to wheat bran for people on special diets.

Pectin – made from fruit and used mainly as a setting agent for jams and a binder in baking with gluten-free flours.

Methylcellulose – manufactured from wood pulp or plant fibres and used as a substitute (cheap) for pectin.

Guar – a kind of gum made from legumes and used to slow down sugar absorption in people with diabetes.

Gum tragacanth – a tree gum used for thickening.

Gum karaya – used as a thickening agent and cheap substitute for gum tragacanth, made from tree gum.

Gum acacia – used in pharmaceutical manufacture in emulsions and to help in granulating, a tree gum.

Glucomannan – almost 100% fibre, made from Konjac seaweed and used as a slimming aid.

Isphagula husk – dried seeds used as a laxative.

Psyllium seeds – used as a laxative.

Oat bran – made from oats.

Fibre in food

The chart that follows shows the percentage of fibre in foods which contain significant amounts of it. These are grains and food made from grains, vegetables and fruit. (Note the absence of high fat foods such as cheese, cream and meat.)

Use the chart sensibly by taking into account just how much of a particular food makes a portion in relation to its fibre content. Parsley, for instance, has a high fibre content but we could not eat more than a few sprigs at a time, whereas cooked carrots do not have such a high fibre content but can be eaten in quite large portions of several ounces. To help you, with this point kept in mind, best fibre foods are indicated by a *.

There is no one standard way of calculating fibre. Some fibres take up water very easily and if weighed wet give a much higher reading than if weighed dry. No one knows this better than the breakfast cereal manufacturer. For this reason figures should only be taken as very approximate, especially if you see them on packaged goods as a claim. 'Contains 15% fibre' if calculated on a wet basis could really mean 'contains only 5% fibre' if calculated on dried basis. (The labelling is unlikely to tell you whether the fibre was wet or dry when the calculations were made.) It is hoped eventually the same method will be used by everyone to standardize fibre calculation. This would mean comparisons would be more accurate than they are at present. However, it will probably need legislation for this improvement to take place.

Fibre content of foods

* *best sources*

Cereals/grains/breads	%
pearl barley (cooked)	2.2
* wheat bran	44.0
* wholewheat flour	9.6
white flour	3.0
brown flour	7.5
* oats (raw)	7.0
boiled white rice	0.8
brown rice	5.5
* low fat soya flour	14.3
* wholewheat bread	8.5
brown bread	5.1
brown bread with wheat germ	4.6
white bread	2.7
All-Bran (also high salt and sugar)	26.7
muesli	7.4
* Puffed Wheat	15.4
* Shredded Wheat	12.3

Biscuits/cakes/pastries
† *made with white flour*

cream crackers†	3.0
* rye crispbread	11.7
Christmas cake†	3.4
Madeira cake†	1.4
sponge†	1.0
mince pies†	2.9
flaky pastry	1.5
shortcrust pastry, cooked	2.4
fruit pie	2.6

Vegetables

* cooked French beans	3.2
* cooked runner beans	3.4
* cooked broad beans	4.2
* boiled butter beans	5.1
* boiled haricot beans	7.4
baked beans in tomato sauce (high salt/sugar)	5.1
* cooked beansprouts	3.0
* raw beetroot	3.1
* cooked beetroot	3.0
* cooked broccoli tops	4.1
cooked Brussels sprouts	2.9
boiled carrots	3.1
* raw carrots	2.9
raw cauliflower	2.1
cooked cauliflower	1.8
raw celery	1.8
raw cucumber	0.4
* boiled leeks	3.9
cooked lentils	3.7
lettuce	1.5
raw mushrooms	2.5
* cooked mushrooms	4.0
spring onions	3.1
parsley	9.1
parsnips	2.5
* fresh boiled peas	5.2
* boiled dried peas	4.8
raw green peppers	0.9
old boiled potatoes	1.0
* new boiled potatoes	2.0
* jacket potatoes incl. skins	2.0

crisps	11.9
radishes	1.0
spinach (boiled)	6.3
* cooked spring greens	3.8
boiled swede	2.8
* canned sweetcorn	5.7
fresh tomatoes	1.5
canned tomatoes	0.9
boiled turnips	2.2
watercress	3.3

Fruit

eating apple	1.5
fresh stewed apricots	1.6
* dried raw apricots	24.0
* stewed dried apricots	8.5
avocado pears	2.0
* bananas	3.4
* stewed blackberries	6.3
cherries	1.7
* stewed blackcurrants	6.8
stewed gooseberries	2.5
black grapes	0.3
white grapes	0.4
grapefruit	0.6
lemons	5.2
melon	1.0 or less
oranges	2.0
* passion fruit	15.9
peaches (dried raw)	14.3
pears	1.7
pineapple	1.2
plums	2.0
* raspberries	7.4
strawberries	2.2
currants	6.5
dates	8.7
* figs (dried raw)	18.5
stewed prunes	7.7
raisins	6.8
sultanas	7.0

Although fibre has come to be associated with 'indigestible', meaning that it will pass through the body unchanged, this is not always so. Some forms of fibre have the ability to swell up, which can considerably affect waste food disposed of by the body.

Probably the most important research made on fibre in our diet concerns the link that has been made with chronic, slowly developed diseases which seem to occur in people who have low levels of fibre in their diets. A particular feature of this kind of diet is the use of very refined products made by removing fibre from foods and, at the same time, vitamins, minerals, protein and, in the case of sugar, water too.

It may be that a diet high in natural fibre can protect against diabetes, gall stones, heart disease, obesity, diverticulitis, cancer of the large bowel, appendicitis, hiatus hernia, varicose veins and haemorrhoids. These complaints are rarely seen in underdeveloped countries. However, we must point out that high fibre is not the only characteristic of the diet in underdeveloped countries. Lower fat levels, less salt, less meat and fish protein, larger amounts of starch and potassium are also features.

The combination of a low-fat diet and oat fibre has been shown to lower blood cholesterol. The trials took place in the USA, with 50g (2oz) oat bran per day per person being used successfully.

One thing that research has shown is that taking fibre by eating unrefined foods seems to be better than eating refined foods from which most of the fibre has been removed *with* separately added bran.

Surveys show that total dietary fibre intakes seem to have halved since 1860 in Britain. This has fallen from 46 g per day when brown flour was used, down to less than 20 g per day for people in higher income groups. The popular use of canned beans and peas in the lower income groups pushes this figure up to 23 g per day. With a suggested level of 35 g per day as a reasonable one, the average person in Britain is not eating enough fibre in the diet. The result of this is difficult to evaluate in terms of effect on health, but people who eat such low levels of fibre exist generally on a selection of foods which are over-refined, with reduced levels of vitamins and minerals too.

The best way of ensuring enough fibre in the diet is to eat more bread of the wholewheat variety, use wholewheat flour for baking and to increase consumption of vegetables and fruits.

Not only does fibre help in cleansing and waste disposal of food from the body but it can play a part in removing harmful toxins as well. Coarse wheat bran is considered to be the best and most effective bran for long term treatment of constipation. It is also used for controlling irritable bowel syndrome, obesity and diabetes.

As always, we can have too much of a good thing and it seems there are adverse effects if too much bran is taken. A sudden change from a low fibre to a high fibre diet can cause diarrhoea and much discomfort from flatulence. Mineral deficiency is another possible effect. In poor countries where diets comprise up to 70% wholewheat bread, small stature, delayed puberty and anaemia caused by zinc deficiency in turn caused by poor absorption of this mineral have been attributed to the high amount of fibre in the diet.

The most effective bran for providing bulk in the diet is probably wheat bran. The best form of this is in wheat flour which has been stoneground, because then the particles of bran are not too finely ground. Fruit and vegetables comprise mainly water, though quite large amounts can be eaten. They are potentially a poor source of fibre, but if large quantities can be eaten they are important as a source of dietary fibre. Dried peas, beans and lentils have good levels of fibre, but these need to be soaked in water before cooking, which really reduces their fibre levels in relation to their weight. For example, dried split peas contain 12% fibre, but after soaking and cooking the level drops to only 5%. Levels of fibre vary from one variety of specific vegetable to another. One type of potato with a thin skin will have less than another variety with a thicker skin. Coconut (desiccated) has a high level of fibre at 24%, but other nuts vary from as little as 5% to 14%. As nuts contain a high proportion of fat they should not really be eaten in large quantities.

Dietary fibre tablets

There is no fibre tablet on the market which contains more than 2% of daily fibre requirements. (Most contain only between 300 to 700 mg of fibre per tablet.) Tablets which contained much more than this would be the size of a walnut! To obtain as much fibre as you need per day, somewhere in the region of 50 tablets would have to be taken every day. The impact of a small number of tablets on the average diet is insignificant, as you can see, with a suggested daily level of 30 g of dietary fibre, and 6 tablets producing only about 4 g. To sum up, fibre tablets seem to be a silly, very expensive and unsuccessful way of adding fibre to a normal diet.

Fibre and slimming

One factor for which slimming dieters crave is the feeling of a full tummy as opposed to hunger pains. The kinds of fibre that readily swell when added to liquid, or vice versa, can be used to fill the stomach, giving a satisfied feeling as if a meal has been eaten, instead of just a little dry fibre and liquid. Glucomannan, isphagula husk, methylcellulose, guar and pectin are the most frequently used fibres for such treatment.

High fibre diets are also used to help slimmers. These usually rely on high fibre foods such as wholewheat bread and beans plus extra fibre in the form of wheat bran (44% fibre). The addition of so much extra bulk to the diet means the dieter feels full after eating and also transit time is increased. The fast passage of food through the body does not leave the digestive system with quite enough time or opportunity to absorb and use all the nutrients in the food. So, some of the food eaten is just not used by the body. By depriving the body of time to totally digest food in this way and by adding food that is indigestible too, you encourage the body to take fat from its stores and convert it to energy. This in turn reduces the size of the fat stores in the body and weight is lost by the dieter.

A sudden switch to much more fibre in the diet can have unpleasant side effects such as flatulence and diarrhoea, so people wishing to lose weight by the high fibre diet method are best advised to increase the fibre in their food gradually to an acceptable level rather than by a swift change. (Diarrhoea can lead to loss of body fluid and potassium.)

Some schools of thought do not accept the extra high fibre slimming method, but prefer a more moderate approach which takes longer to achieve weight loss but, from a nutritional point of view, is much more sensible.

□ *Carbohydrates*

A very important function of food is to provide the body with energy. The foods that are richest in carbohydrate are starches and sugars.

Plants can store up energy for future use in the form of starch. They are able to do this by forming sugar in their leaves, converting the sugar to starch and storing it in other parts of their structure – in roots, stems, seeds or tubers. Not surprisingly, plants provide us with a substantial part of the carbohydrate in our diet.

After carbohydrate undergoes the process of digestion it is converted mainly to glucose. This is found in the juices of plants and fruit as well the blood of live animals. Fructose (fruit sugar) is found in fruit and vegetables as well as honey and is very sweet. Sucrose is less sweet and is processed from cane and beet and is also found in small quantities in fruit and vegetables. Chemically speaking it is a combination of fructose and glucose. The white, refined sugar we know as 'caster' or 'granulated' sugar is pure sucrose. To make it, large amounts of fibre are refined out from the cane or beet, leaving behind a pure form of carbohydrate.

Although we need carbohydrate in our diet to give us energy, it is all too easy to eat too much of it in the form of sugar, which has a delightful taste to most people. The following chart shows the levels of carbohydrate in foods common in our diet. Those with a combination of starch and sugar such as cakes and biscuits are probably the worst types of food for health. The healthiest high carbohydrate foods are those which contain a fair amount of fibre as well. So, wholewheat bread is a more valuable food than sponge cake. Foods with the lowest levels of carbohydrate are eggs, meat, fish (all high protein foods) and fats and oils.

Carbohydrate content of edible foods
in grammes per 100g (or %)

* *best sources for health*	
pearl barley	83.6
wheat germ	44.7
wheat bran	26.8
cornflour (maize flour)	92.0
* wholewheat flour	67.8
white flour	74.8
self-raising flour	77.5
* boiled pasta	25.2
oat porridge	8.2
* boiled rice	86.8
rye flour	75.9
soya flour	23.5
* wholewheat bread	41.8
brown bread	44.7
white bread	49.7
All-Bran	43.0
cornflakes	85.1
* muesli	66.2
* Shredded Wheat	67.9
* rye crispbread	70.6
plain digestives	66.0
rich fruit cake	58.3
shortcrust pastry	55.8
fruit pie	56.7
milk pudding	20.4
treacle tart	61.3
cow's milk	4.7
dried skimmed milk	52.8
butter	*trace*
double cream	2.0

most cheeses	*trace*
natural yoghurt	6.2
fruit yoghurt	17.9
eggs	*trace*
oils/fats	tr. or 0
meat/poultry	tr. or 0
liver	0.6 to 2.2
grilled sausages	15.2
fish/molluscs	0
French beans	1.1
broad beans	7.1
* boiled butter beans	17.1
* boiled haricot beans	16.6
baked beans in tomato sauce	10.3
boiled beetroot	9.9
boiled broccoli tops	1.6
Brussels sprouts	1.7
raw red cabbage	3.5
old carrots	5.4
boiled cauliflower	0.8
cucumber	1.8
boiled leeks	4.6
* boiled lentils	17.0
lettuce	1.2
mushrooms	0
raw onion	5.2
boiled peas	7.7
* boiled split peas	21.9
raw green pepper	2.2
* old potatoes (baked)	25.0
chips	37.3
spinach	1.4
boiled sweetcorn	22.8
tomatoes	2.8
watercress	0.7
apples	11.9
apricots	6.7
bananas	19.2
blackberries	6.4
cherries	11.9
stewed dried figs	34.3
dates	63.9
grapes	15.5 to 16.1

grapefruit	5.3
melon	5.3
oranges	8.5
peaches	9.1
pears	10.6
pineapple	11.6
stewed prunes with sugar	26.5
raisins	64.4
raspberries	5.6
strawberries	6.2
sultanas	64.7
almonds	4.3
brazils	4.1
hazel nuts	6.8
coconut	3.7
peanuts	8.6
peanut butter	13.1
walnuts	5.0
glucose	84.7
demerara sugar	104.5
white sugar	105.0
black treacle	67.2
honey	74.4
jam/marmalade	69.0
marzipan	49.2
mincemeat	62.1
boiled sweets	87.3
chocolate bars	58.3 to 66.5
toffees	71.1
wines and spirits	*very low*

□*Fats and oils in our food*

It is important to know about the role of fats/oils in the diet as some vitamins are what is called 'fat-soluble'. They are taken into the body as part of fats/oils and the basic ones are vitamins A, D, E, F and K.

The fats and oils available to us in our diet come in many forms. For baking and spreading we can use butter or margarine. For cooking we have a whole array of products ranging from lard to oils extracted from beans, nuts and seeds. Some are from animal sources and others are from vegetables. Many of the foods we eat comprise partly fat, such as meat, milk, nuts, cheese and eggs.

Fat content of some foods (average)
in grammes per 100 g

Fats/oils	%
cooking oil	99.9
lard, dripping	99.3
margarine	85.3
butter	82.5
'low fat' spread	40.5

Meat	
bacon	27.0 – 44.8
pork	6.9 – 26.3
lamb	8.1 – 29.0
beef	4.4 – 28.8
calf's liver	7.3
chicken	5.4
turkey	1.4 – 6.9
veal	2.7
fried sausages	18.0
corned beef	12.1
ham	5.1

Fish	
fatty fish	
herring	15.1
kipper	11.4
mackerel	8.3
canned salmon	8.2
canned sardines	13.6
non-fatty fish	
plaice	1.9
sole	0.9
cod	1.1
haddock	0.8

Dairy produce	
single cream	21.2
double cream	48.2
Cheddar cheese	33.5

Stilton cheese	40.0
Edam cheese	22.9
eggs	10.9
milk (whole)	3.8
skimmed milk (dried)	1.3

Grain products

oats	8.7
wholewheat bread	2.7
white bread	1.7
wholewheat flour	2.0
white flour	1.2
spaghetti	1.0
rice	1.0

Vegetables

potatoes, green vegetables, peas, beans, carrots etc.	*trace*

Fruit

avocado pears	11 to 39 *depending on season*
olives	8.8
all other fruits	*trace*

Nuts

desiccated coconut	62.0
brazil nuts	61.5
almonds	53.5
walnuts	51.5
peanuts	49.0

The terms used to describe fats will probably be familiar to you – saturated, polyunsaturated (or unsaturated). They tend to be misleading as no fat or oil comprises just one of these, but a mixture of saturated, mono-unsaturated and polyunsaturated fats, plus a few more obscure ones too. Fats and oils are loosely described by the kind of fat which features most in their composition. For example, we refer to certain margarines as being 'polyunsaturated'. Although they do indeed contain a high proportion of polyunsaturated fat, mono-unsaturated fat and saturated fats are also present in them.

A myth prevails, and this is partly due to advertising, that all animal fats are saturated and all vegetable oils are polyunsaturated. This is quite wrong. Coconut and palm oils are both very high in saturated fat and yet are vegetable oils. To explain the composition of

fats and oils more clearly here is a chart which shows how much
saturated fat and how much polyunsaturated fat there is in the basic
fats and oils we use in our food. (Note the percentages added together
will not equal 100 as there are other fats present too. To avoid confusion these are not listed on the chart.)

Approximate saturated and polyunsaturated fat in fats and oils etc.

as percentages

food	saturated	polyunsaturated
cream, butter	61	3
suet	58	1
lard	44	10
hard margarine	38	16
vegetable oil, hard block	38	16
polyunsaturated margarine	25	55
egg yolk	38	11
ice cream	67	3
olive oil	15	12
coconut oil	80	2
palm oil	49	9
groundnut oil (peanut)	20.5	30
soya oil	15	60
sunflower seed oil	14	52
safflower seed oil	11	76
maize oil (corn)	17	52

Ideally our diet should contain both saturated and unsaturated
fats. The main sources of fat in our diet are milk, cheese, cream,
yoghurt, meat and meat products, fish and fish products, cooking oils,
nuts, seeds, butter and margarines. By eating a varied diet without too
much animal fat, a reasonable balance can be maintained between the
two kinds of fat.

Visible and invisible fats

Some fats are easily identified in our diet: e.g. the fat on meat,
either in white layers or 'marbled areas'; spreads such as butter
and margarine; and cooking oils. These are called 'visible fats' for
obvious reasons. Other forms of fats are called 'invisible fats' as
we cannot readily see them in foods: e.g. avocado pear has quite a
high fat content. Milk, yoghurt, nuts all contain fat.

Fats are a very concentrated source of energy. They can be used immediately for energy or stored in our bodies until required. Overweight people have overlarge fat stores. The fat builds up in layers all over the body, under the skin, around the organs of the body and even as a lining in the arteries.

High fat foods are very satisfying to eat as they stay in the stomach for quite a while. Most fats also taste nice too. Would we eat cream if it didn't taste so good? The variety of tastes in fats is amazing. Look at the vast selection of cheeses that can be made from milk, each with its unique personality – hundreds of different kinds.

Different fatty acids in each fat or oil help to give fats and oils their own particular characteristics. While saturated fats are reasonably stable, polyunsaturated fats are less so and will gradually turn rancid if in contact with the air. This alters both the colour, which darkens, and the taste, which can become most unpleasant. By a process called 'hydrogenation', manufacturers are able to turn unsaturated fatty acids into saturated fatty acids to make them keep better.

There are many saturated fatty acids but the most important one is probably *palmitic acid*, which features largely in the composition of animal fats, especially lard and suet – the 'hard' fats. *Stearic, lauric* and *myristic acids* are three other important saturated fatty acids.

Unsaturated fatty acids of importance are:

Oleic acid – found in all fats, but in high concentrations in olive oil.

Linoleic acid – found in pork in small amounts and in some other animal fats. It is found in larger amounts in seeds oils, e.g. maize (corn) oil, soya oil.

Linolenic acid – found in vegetable oils in small amounts. The oil with the most significant amount is linseed oil.

Gamma–Linolenic acid – found in the seeds of the evening primrose, borage leaves and in spirulina. It can also be made by the body by converting linolenic acid.

Arachidonic acid – found in some animal fats, but only in small amounts. It can be made in the body by converting linolenic acid. (See Vitamin F for further information, page 102.)

You may have heard the term *Essential Fatty Acids* or EFAs as they are sometimes called. These are linoleic, linolenic, gamma –linolenic acid and arachidonic acid. They belong to the F family of vitamins and, as their name suggests, they are essential.

There is a tendency in the Western diet, particularly among affluent people, to consume too much fat. One of the causes of heart disease can be hardening of the arteries (atherosclerosis). Although much controversy rages about this, it is thought that the increased cholesterol concentrations in the blood frequently found in overweight people may be partly to blame. The link between a diet with a high proportion of saturated animal fat and high cholesterol has not yet been proved to the satisfaction of all scientists. However, commonsense should indicate that although it has not yet been quite proved satisfactorily, making sure that we eat a diet that will produce lower levels of cholesterol is not harmful and can be enjoyed as a possible preventive measure against heart disease. It has been proved that it is possible to lower cholesterol by modifying the diet by taking less fat altogether and making sure that over half of the fat taken is unsaturated.

□ *Cholesterol*

There is much confusion about cholesterol, which is not actually a fat but a fat-like substance called a lipid. It is found only in animal products and here is a chart to give you some idea of just how much cholesterol some foods contain.

Cholesterol in foods
in mg per 100 g, approx 4 oz

Grain products	mg
rich fruit cake	50
sponge cake (with fat)	130
bread and butter pudding	100
dairy ice cream	21
non-dairy ice cream	11
milk pudding	15
pancakes	65
Yorkshire pudding	70
Milk and eggs	
whole, fresh cow's milk	14
longlife	14
dried whole milk	120
dried skimmed milk	18
salted butter	230
single cream	66
double cream	140
whipping cream	100

Camembert type cheese	72
Cheddar type cheese	70
Blue Vein type	88
Parmesan	90
Stilton	120
cottage cheese	13
cream cheese	94
low fat natural yoghurt	7
egg yolks	1260
egg white	0
boiled eggs (white and yolk)	450

Fats/oils

beef dripping	60
lard	70
shredded suet	74
vegetable oils	*trace*

Meat and offal

fried bacon, lean and fat	80
beef	82
lamb	110
pork	110
chicken, roast	
light meat	74
dark meat	120
roast duck	160
turkey,	
light meat	49
dark meat	100
calves' and lambs' brains	2200
fried lambs' kidneys	610
fried calves' liver	330
fried lamb's liver	400
corned beef	85
ham	33
tongue	110
liver sausage	120
fried beef sausages	42
grilled beef sausages	42
pork sausages, fried or grilled	53
fried beefburgers	68
pork pie	52
suet pastry	125
beef stew	30

Fish

baked cod	60
steamed haddock	75
steamed plaice	90
grilled herring	80
fried mackerel	90
canned salmon	90
canned sardines	100
lobster	150
prawns	200
scampi	110
mussels	100
fried herring roe	500

Note that all these foods are from animal sources, not vegetable sources.

Vegetarian dishes are usually lower in cholesterol than ones which contain meat and fish. However, too many eggs and too much cheese, milk and cream can soon bring the levels up again. Vegan diets are cholesterol-free as vegans do not eat any kind of product from an animal. This does not mean that vegans have no cholesterol in their bodies, because they do. It can be synthesized mainly in the liver and in the intestines.

Sources of fat-soluble vitamins

Vitamins A and D are found in fish oils. We are able to make vitamin D in our bodies from sunshine. Other sources are egg yolk, milk, fish and fish bones. In Britain vitamins A and D are added to margarine. As beta carotene, vitamin A can be obtained from green or yellow vegetables, e.g. carrots and spinach. Vitamin E is found in butter, vegetables with dark green leaves, eggs, fruit, nuts, vegetable oils and wheat germ. Vitamin F is found in safflower oil, sunflower oil, corn and soya oils, wheat germ, evening primrose seeds, borage and fish oils. Vitamin K is available from vegetables with green leaves, safflower oil, yoghurt, oats.

□*Protein*

Protein is needed for growth and repair. If we take in more than we need, the surplus can be converted into energy. No one food is pure protein and the foods which provide a good source of protein

as well as other nutrients are meat, fish, milk, cheese and eggs –
all animal proteins – and nuts, peas and beans (legumes), wheat,
maize and rice (cereals). Green leafy vegetables are poor sources
and root vegetables such as carrots and potatoes contain only very
little in the way of protein. However, some low protein foods can
be eaten in large quantities, e.g. potatoes, and this makes them
quite a good source of protein from a practical point of view.

Here is a table which shows comparative protein levels of
some foods.

Average protein content of some foods
in grammes per 100 g (or %)

Cereals/grains (and products)

wheat germ	26.5
wheat bran	14.1
wholewheat flour	13.2
raw oats	12.4
porridge	1.4
boiled pasta	4.3
boiled rice	2.2
low fat soya flour	45.3
wholewheat bread	8.8
brown bread plus wheat germ	9.7
white bread	7.8
muesli	12.9
Shredded Wheat	10.6
starch reduced wheat crispbread	45.3
rye crispbread	9.4
rich fruit cake	3.7
sponge cake with fat	6.4
doughnuts	6.0
shortcrust pastry	6.9
scones	7.5
bread and butter pudding	6.1
egg custard	5.8
fruit pie with pastry top	2.0
jelly	1.4
rice pudding	3.4
pancakes	6.1
Yorkshire pudding	6.8

Milk and milk products

fresh whole milk	3.3
dried skimmed milk	36.4
made up	3.4
butter	0.4
single cream	2.4
double cream	1.5
Camembert type cheese	22.8
Cheddar type cheese	26.0
Blue Vein type cheese	23.0
Parmesan	35.1
Edam	24.4
Stilton	25.6
cottage cheese	13.6
natural yoghurt	5.0

Eggs

boiled eggs (2 average)	12.3
egg white	9.0
scrambled eggs	10.5

Meat

grilled back bacon, lean and fat	25.3
grilled streaky, lean and fat	24.5
cooked, lean minced beef	23.1
grilled rumpsteak, lean and fat	27.3
stewed steak, lean and fat	30.9
loin lamb chops, grilled, lean only	27.8
roast leg of lamb, lean only	29.4
roast leg of pork, lean only	30.7
roast chicken, lean only	24.8
roast turkey, light meat	29.8
fried lamb's liver	22.9
corned beef	26.9
ham	18.4
sausages	10.6
beef stew	9.6

Fish

baked cod	21.4
fried haddock	21.4
plaice fried in batter	15.8
grilled herring	20.4
fried mackerel	21.5
canned salmon	20.3

sardines	23.7
tuna	22.8
prawns	8.6
scampi	12.2
mussels	17.2
fish cakes	10.5

Vegetables

asparagus	3.4
French beans	0.8
runner beans	1.9
broad beans	4.1
boiled butter beans	7.1
baked beans in tomato sauce	5.1
broccoli tops	3.3
red cabbage	1.7
carrots	0.8
cauliflower	1.9
celery	0.9
cucumber	0.6
boiled leeks	1.8
cooked lentils	7.6
lettuce	1.0
fried mushrooms	2.2
fried onions	1.8
raw parsley	5.2
boiled peas	5.0
boiled dried split peas	8.3
green peppers	0.9
old boiled potatoes	1.4
jacket potatoes	2.1
chips	3.8
radishes	1.0
boiled spinach	5.1
spring greens	1.7
swedes	0.9
canned sweetcorn	2.9
tomatoes	0.9
turnips	0.7
watercress	2.9

Fruits
These are very low in protein, being around 1% or less. Dried fruits such as apricots, figs and prunes have slightly higher concentrations of protein, but none is as high as 4%.

Proteins consist of chains of *amino acids*. The arrangement of these minute components varies a good deal as there are more than twenty amino acids known to exist in body proteins and the chains may number hundreds or even thousands of amino acids.

There are two main types of amino acids – *essential* and *non-essential*. (Don't be misled by the term 'non-essential'. It refers to very necessary amino acids and the term merely means that they don't need to be taken into the body in food because the body can actually make them.) The 'essential' amino acids *must* be acquired by the body from the food it takes in as the body is unable to make them in large enough quantities for health. All proteins contain some of the non-essential amino acids. Certain of the amino acids in food provide the body with the materials to make the range of non-essential amino acids it needs.

There are eight amino acids that seem to be essential for adults – isoleucine, leucine, lysine, methionine, phenylalanine, threonine, tryptophan and valine. Children who are growing quickly also need an extra one – histidine. Other amino acids are widespread in proteins. You will see a selection listed in the section on amino acids (see pages 139–163).

Our bodies have no way of storing a surplus of amino acids until they are required so we need to keep up a regular supply of them. Because different sources of protein offer different levels of the various amino acids some foods are more valuable to us in terms of amino acids than others. As you would expect, animal proteins are most like those of man and provide the most useful assortment of amino acids. Those available from vegetable sources present quite different combinations and are not as valuable to man as animal proteins. However, by combining several different vegetable proteins, a better balance of amino acids can be obtained. What is lacking in one vegetable protein is then made up by another and so on. You can see how important it is to eat a mixed diet so that a variety of proteins is taken in food. The combination of animal and vegetable proteins is an excellent one and the old idea of a meal being 'meat and two veg' is a sound nutritional one.

It is important for vegetarians and vegans to eat a good variety of vegetables and grains to make sure of enough of the essential amino acids that meat eaters normally obtain from animal protein.

Animals present a very expensive form of protein as they need to convert plant protein to muscle (animal protein). Their process for doing this is not very efficient and this is one reason why animal protein is so expensive. To make cheaper forms of protein available, processes for extracting protein from beans and plants have been developed. TVP [textured vegetable protein] is one such example, and to make such products closer to meat for food value, supplements are added such as thiamin, riboflavin, vitamin B12 etc.

The Amino Acids section (pages 139ff.) will tell you the best uses and sources of particular amino acids. Very little is known about many of them and new research is being carried out all the time.

■3   Sensible diet

□*Dietary balance and essential nutrients*

One of the most hackneyed phrases of the anti-vitamin lobby is the cry that no one eating a 'balanced diet' can be deficient in vitamins and minerals. The argument continues that since we are, at least in Britain and the Western World, supposedly better fed than ever before in history, there is absolutely no way there can be any general health problems relating to vitamin deficiencies. As soon as these people are asked to give examples of individuals following the balanced diet and to explain how those who constantly gorge on junk food, sweets as well as on very fatty, salty and sugary foods can possibly have a balanced diet, they seem to lapse into silence!

The real picture is quite different. Hardly anyone is eating an ideal balanced diet. As an example, take babies. Baby foods and breast milk substitutes can lead to nutritional problems, probably laying a foundation for a future of potentially poor health for adults. Human milk substitutes prepared from cow's milk provide babies with many nutrient imbalances if it is assumed that breast milk is the standard which should be copied. Not only are the vitamin and mineral balance different, but because cow's milk proteins have a different balance of amino acids from human milk protein, other important elements are wrongly balanced too. (Amino acids are discussed on pages 139–163.)

The human body is a very resilient machine and may well be able to adjust to wide variations of diet. Certain precautionary positive steps on the part of each person could make things better. A move towards a natural style of diet with reduction of processed and junk foods would provide us all with something nearer to a balance, the need for which we have inherited over countless generations.

Whilst the ingestion of junk and processed foods may produce deficiencies of essential nutrients, in rare circumstances some

Chart showing the differences between mature human milk and regular breast-milk substitutes

per 100 ml (– indicates no figure available or inappropriate)

Nutrient	mature human milk	cow's milk based substitute		soya milk based substitute	
			% difference		% difference
protein g	1.3	1.8	+38	2.9	+123
fat (total) g*	4.1	2.4	−41	2.6	−37
carbohydrate g	7.2	8.3	+15	8.0	+11
sodium mg	14	31	+121	40	+186
potassium mg	58	79	+36	105	+81
calcium mg	34	65	+91	115	+238
magnesium mg	3	—	—	9.4	+213
phosphorus mg	14	53	+279	94	+571
iron mcg***	70	650	+829	800	+1043
copper mcg	40	38	−5	58	+45
zinc mcg	280	310	+11	430	+54
retinol vitamin A mcg	60	95	+58	90	+50
vitamin D mcg***	0.025	1	+3,900	1.2	+4700
vitamin B1 mcg	20	38	+90	81	+305
vitamin B2 mcg	30	51	+70	120	+300
vitamin B3 mcg**	220	640	+191	610	+177
vitamin C mg	3.7	6.2	+68	6.6	+78
vitamin E mcg	340	450	+32	1080	+218
vitamin B6 mcg	10	32	+220	48	+380
vitamin B12 mcg	*trace* (0.1)	0.13	—	0.12	—
folic acid mcg	5	3.1	−38	6	+20
pantothenic acid mcg	250	220	−12	240	−4
biotin mcg	0.7	0.95	+36	1.71	+144
manganese mcg	*trace*	3.1	—	17	—
chloride	37.5	58	+55	75	+100
choline	8.9	—	—	4.7	−47

* Total fat given, but human milk is approximately 50% saturated, 40% mono-unsaturated and 10% polyunsaturated including gamma linolenic acid, which is not present in any of these substitutes.

** Niacin (nicotinic acid) is the form in human milk. Nicotinamide is used in the substitutes.

*** Considerable fortification is carried out to produce these levels in the substitute.

diets could provide other problems. Fad slimming diets are particularly hazardous in throwing nutrient balances into chaos. It is always wise to take a comprehensive vitamin and mineral supplement concentrate when following one of these diets.

Some years ago there was a grapefruit diet widely promoted – this could lead to excess vitamin C and result in over-acidifying the body. Liver as a staple meat can produce excesses of vitamin A with resultant jaundice. (Polar bear liver has so much vitamin A present that over-indulgence in it can be fatal, as Arctic Circle explorers found to their cost.) This does not mean that either grapefruit or polar bear liver is in any way dangerous if eaten in sensible amounts – it is the lack of balance that is the problem. Even water in excess will be toxic – if you drink so much water that your stomach is always full, you will be unable to eat any food and could consequently die.

Eat a good mixed diet of fresh ingredients and your body will have the fuel and micronutrients it requires to maintain good health. Even a balanced diet can be improved with supplemental insurance and this will be discussed later.

□A sensible diet

The key to a sensible diet is to eat the right mixture of foods to ensure sufficient nutrients, but it should also be related to the kind of life you lead. It is pointless, for instance, to eat enough food for a lumberjack if you are only an office worker. If you are elderly you do not need the same kind of diet as a growing child, and so on.

While eating food is an activity vital for life itself, it is wise not to eat just any old food, but to choose a little more carefully for best results regarding your health.

In 1983, what is known as the NACNE Report was published in Britain (National Advisory Committee on Nutritional Education). This represented a milestone in nutritional thinking as it suggested new and lower levels of fat, salt and sugar in our daily diet but more fibre, fresh foods, vegetables and fruit. This is mainly because research showed that most of us eat too much processed food, allowing too much fat, sugar and salt and far too little fibre in our diet. We don't eat enough bread but we eat far too many biscuits, cakes and pastries. When we do eat bread it is usually the wrong kind (white), with too little fibre. We eat too much meat (including the fat) and not enough fish. We salt our food out of habit rather than need, making sure we take too much. We use the frying pan and deep fryer too often. Far too many of us are overweight, which is not surprising in view of the alarming amount of sugar we consume per head – in jam, in beverages and confectionery. By the time we have reached forty most of us will be suffering from at least one Western type of disease. What a depressing picture of the average person today! If you feel you might fit this description regarding your eating habits, here's how you can start to improve your diet immediately:

Butter: cut down by one third.

Fatty meats such as pork, beef, mutton and lamb: cut down by one third.

Liver: double your consumption.

Increase *poultry* consumption by half again.

Cut your consumption of *sausages* by half.

Fish: double or even treble consumption.

Jams, sugar and sweets: cut these by half.

Potatoes: double the amount.

Fresh fruit and vegetables: double the amount.

Dried beans and pulses: eat three times as many.

Bread: double the amount and go over to largely wholewheat.

Cakes, pastries and biscuits: cut by one third.

Margarines and other fats: cut by one third.

Change to *low-fat milk* instead of whole milk.

Oils: change to polyunsaturated oil.

Salt: cut right down on salt in cooking. Don't add salt at the table.

Cereals: change to wholewheat, without sugar and salt.

To give you some idea of what your diet should look like, the (approximate) NACNE report recommendations for one person's food intake for one week are shown in chart form.

Suggested food intake for one person per week based on the recommendations of the NACNE Report

Milk (preferably skimmed or semi-skimmed) *2 pints (1 litre)*

Eggs
  2½

Fats/Oils
  margarine (polyunsaturated) *under 3 oz (75 g)*
  cheeses (preferably low fat) *4 oz (100 g)*
  butter *under 2 oz (50 g)*
  unsaturated oil (preferably safflower or sunflower) *9 fluid oz (270 ml)*

Sensible diet

Vegetables
potatoes 3½ lbs (1¾ kg)
frozen vegetables 3 oz (75 g)
fresh greens and other vegetables 2½ lbs (1¼ kg)
canned vegetables 10 oz (280 g)

Meat
lean only from *approx 2 lbs (1 kg)* total weight before trimming,
boning and cooking
beef 4½ oz (120 g)
liver 1½ oz (40 g)
lamb 2½ oz (60 g)
bacon/ham 4 oz (100 g)
sausages 1½ oz (40 g)
pork 2½ oz (60 g)
poultry 10 oz (280 g)
other meat products 4½ oz (120 g)

Fish
about 10 oz (280 g) total weight before filleting

Fruit
over *2 lbs (1 kg)* fresh fruit
canned fruit (preferably low sugar) 2 oz (50 kg)
dried fruit and nuts 8 oz (250 g)

Rice/Pasta/Noodles
1 lb (½ kg) (preferably wholewheat pasta and brown rice)

Bread
approx 3 lbs (1½ kg) total
wholewheat 1¼ lbs (over ½ kg)
white 12 oz (320 g)
brown 12 oz (320 g)
other breads 4 oz (100 g)

Biscuits
about 4 oz (100 g)

Flour
(preferably wholewheat) *about 6 oz (150 kg)*

Cereals
(breakfast) 8 oz (250 g)

Cakes/Buns/Pastry
under 3 oz (under 75 g)

Pulses
(dried beans, lentils, peas) 1½ oz (40 g)

Beverages
½ oz (15 g)

Sugar
  5 oz (125 g)
Jam/Marmalade
  4 oz (100 g)
Other Foods
  about 9 oz (270 g)

If you would like to improve on this regime still further, we suggest the following:
Cut out sausages and other meat products unless made at home.
Cut down more on sugar and meat.
Use more wholewheat bread and cut right down on the white and brown.
Use wholegrain pasta and rice.
Omit the canned fruit and vegetables. Increase the fresh ones.

If you are a *vegetarian* omit the fish and meat. Increase pulses, nuts and eggs, low fat milk and low fat cheeses to make sure of enough protein. Use soya protein instead of part of the meat allowance.

Either of these diets should yield enough nutrients for a healthy regime. Notice the large amount of fresh vegetables and fruit. If these are eaten in raw form, where appropriate, then so much the better. The minimum of processed foods should be used in order to obtain the maximum vitamins and minerals from fresh foods. Cooked foods should not be *over* cooked. Steamed or stir/fry vegetables are preferable to boiled ones. Jacket potatoes are better than peeled, boiled or roasted ones, if the skin is also eaten. New potatoes are best boiled in their skins. Only the type of person undergoing tremendous physical exercise or heavy labouring should be likely to need to add salt to cooking and at table, unless they are under medical supervision for an illness requiring more salt (sodium).

□*Bread*

The bread we buy at the baker's and supermarket is not made in the same way as bread baked at home. Shop bread may be several days old before it is even put on the shelf and will probably have several additives – colouring, something to make it rise well, something to make it keep for several days, plenty of salt and mysterious 'improvers'. The very best kind of bread can be made at home from simple and good ingredients. In the right conditions it will keep for several days and can be eaten plain, toasted, used as crumbs for cooking, for croutons, bread and butter pudding, fruit charlotte and other dishes. Crumbs can also be used as a meat extender in rissoles. There is therefore no need to waste homemade bread after having taken the trouble to make it.

Here is a very simple kind of bread. Make it with stoneground, wholewheat flour and it will have up to three times as much valuable cereal fibre as its white counterpart.

Simple Bread   *makes 3 small loaves*

1 oz (25 g) fresh yeast,
1 teaspoon sugar,
2lb (900 g) wholewheat flour (stoneground),
just under 1 pint (500 ml) warm water,
1 tablespoon sunflower oil
(salt is not necessary, but, if you wish to use it, ½ to 1 level teaspoon is ample)

Method   Put the yeast and sugar into a small basin. Mix to a cream and add 3 tablespoons warm water. Stir well and then leave in a warm place. As the yeast begins to 'work', the mixture will become frothy. It should be ready to use after about 10 to 15 minutes.

Put the flour into a warm mixing bowl. Add the oil and stir with a fork to distribute it. Make a well in the centre and pour in the frothy yeast. Pour in more of the warm water and stir with a wooden spoon to make a very rough dough. Add more water and mix it in until you can actually stir the dough. Put a clean tea towel over the bowl and leave it in a warm place to rise. (This is called 'proving'.) After 30 to 40 minutes the dough should have risen well and look both wet and light. It should also have a sour, yeasty smell. Now work the dough by hand, sprinkling in more flour to make it drier and heavier. You will find, as you start to work it, that it will collapse back to a smaller amount. Mix to a sticky lump and then turn it out on to a floured worktop. Now the dough must be kneaded. Sprinkle the dough as well as your hands with flour. Press and push the heel of each hand on to the dough, making it flatter and stretching it. With the fingertips fold it back on to itself and begin again. Keep the dough in one large lump and with a few minutes' effort you should have a smooth dough without any air holes. (You can cut it with a knife to see, if you are not sure.) Divide the dough into 3 equally sized pieces and shape into fat sausages. Grease 3x1lb loaf tins and place dough in each one. Press the dough into the corners of the tins with the knuckles. Again, leave to rise in a warm place, but this time uncovered. Preheat the oven at Gas Mark 7 (220°C/425°F). When the loaves have risen to the top of the tins, but before the dough begins to crack, put into the oven on the centre shelf. Bake for 30 to 35 minutes. Turn out of the tins immediately and cool on a wire rack.

☐ *Common causes of nutrient deficiency*

In developing countries of the world famine is still the largest single cause of malnutrition. Plagues of pests, drought or flood leads to crop failure and there simply is not enough food to go round. In the developed countries there is plenty of food – more than enough to go round. In spite of this people still suffer from deficiencies for many reasons, e.g:

1 Poor quality food due to overprocessing and long storage.

2 Poverty.

3 Ignorance. The average person's knowledge of suitable diet and nutrition for their particular lifestyle is extremely poor.

4 Anorexia. Boredom, depression and inertia tend to decrease the appetite. Elderly, retired people, especially those living alone, are prone to this, but it is also becoming widespread among young girls who carry the slimming obsession to extremes.

5 Dental problems. Being able to chew food properly is a necessary part of digestion. Missing teeth, dental caries, gum disorders and mouth infections account for some poor eating habits, particularly in the elderly. If eating becomes painful instead of pleasurable, then food is avoided.

6 Poor digestion. This is sometimes caused by absorption defect diseases which are not always severe enough for diagnosis. Some people, on the other hand, suffer from poor digestion. Flatulence, heartburn and indigestion are common ailments in modern Britain, as the sales of indigestion remedies testify.

7 Chronic disease. People suffering from chronic disease need the very best nutrition. All too often loss of appetite and poor care result in poor nutrition.

8 Aging. Like everything else, our bodies eventually wear out. Elderly people may not be able to secrete as much gastric juice or produce enough enzymes for digestion as they did when younger.

9 Apathy. Lack of energy, incentive and imagination can lead to loss of interest in food. Preparing proper meals

becomes too much trouble, resulting in a poor standard of nutrition. Shopping, with the advent of the supermarket and self service store, has become more difficult compared with the days when orders were delivered to people's homes. Some people would rather go without food than face shopping for it, particularly those living in cities.

10 Fads. Slimming, imaginary or real food allergies, religious or conscience cults can lead to peculiar dietary balances. Combined with poor knowledge of nutrition this can lead to deficiencies.

Other facets of deficiencies of nutrients are discussed in more detail, where appropriate, throughout the book.

□*Nutrient Deficiency Assessments (NDAs)*

One of the most frequently asked questions is, 'How do I know what vitamins I need?' Enquirers then give details of their present health problems.

Any answer must start by ensuring that the person is already taking a balanced, naturally based diet. In most cases, if this is not already being followed, sound advice on diet can often bring about great health improvements, quickly. We usually recommend taking a comprehensive general supplement (multivitamin/ mineral) and at the same time changing the diet, but with the advice that the supplement be discontinued when the improved diet is well established.

If people are leading the sort of life which makes a good diet, at all times, almost impossible to achieve, then diet supplementation insurance is no bad thing. The groups we have in mind include executives rushing about the world in aeroplanes, trains and cars, habitually using mass catering facilities; housewives trying to cope with job and family; elderly folk who find cooking and food preparation a bore; children eating no breakfast and trying to survive on poor school meals or junk snacks; teenagers rushing meals to go to the disco; working adults relying for a main midday meal on sandwich bars, pub snacks and staff canteens.

Several books have appeared since 1980 which attempt to help guide readers to their best supplementary regime. These are all basically the same, but people have become muddled because of fairly minor differences between the recommendations. A deviation of as little as just 100 mg vitamin C between regimes will, not surprisingly, confuse lay people.

Our advice is clear – no one regime or supplementation will

suit everybody. If you believe you are at risk of deficiency because of diet and lifestyle, find a good, natural comprehensive supplement that suits you. There are several which are formulated for general groups and these may make your search less arduous. Do not worry if you have to try several before you find the one that you feel is best for yourself. There are considerable differences between brands. Use your chosen one regularly and top up with vitamin C in winter.

Specific health problems can be helped by further refinement of the diet and supplemental regimes. Items like extra of particular vitamins or a specific amino acid can be added, but the basic regime of a good diet and chosen general supplement should still form the foundation of the system. Nutritional treatments are holistic and no 'wonder drugs' exist, although the addition of just one concentrate to an already correct basic regime can show immediate results. It is the whole system which is right for you, not just the last item which needed the rest before it could do its work.

Laboratory tests as well as personalized systems from books are available to help you in your search for the right nutritional regime. The tests, like the personalized system, only provide you with extra information in your search and no single test will guarantee results. Blood tests, hair tests and computerized tests based on questionnaires may all be helpful. However, these tests are still considered to be controversial or unproven. Often their expense is not justified unless you are under a professional nutritionist who is qualified to interpret the results. Some simpler computerized tests are now becoming available but we still feel that a degree of qualified advice should accompany the results.

■4　What are micronutrients?

□ *What are vitamins?*

The word vitamin has in general conversation lost its original meaning. Most lay people understand vitamins as substances needed to stay alive and vital, and found in food. In addition, pills or capsules found in colourfully labelled bottles or boxes at the chemists and with somewhat mysterious names in health stores, are also called vitamins by many people. Usually these products are actually labelled as dietary supplements or tonics.

Even in scientific terms, the word 'vitamin' is not clearly defined. Originally the term meant an essential natural chemical substance only found in micro-quantities in food. This was to contrast them with substances like proteins, fats and carbohydrates which were known to be needed in large amounts in food. The maximum amount originally thought to be needed for a substance to qualify as a vitamin was about 100 mg per day. Then it was discovered that other substances were essential but needed in quantities of well over 100 mg daily, e.g. essential fatty acids. It was also found that certain vitamins could be made naturally within the body and their intake in food was not vital.

In the 1930s and 1940s there was great activity in organic chemistry, with research laboratories everywhere concentrating efforts on trying to find new drugs and vitamins to patent. This led to great confusion and the results are still with us today.

Everyone will have noticed that the vitamins are usually identified in two ways: either by a letter of the alphabet, perhaps followed by a number or rarely another letter; or as a more complicated chemical name, for example vitamin A is also known as retinol and vitamin B12 as cyanocobalamin. Even more confusing to many people is the fact that not all vitamins are recognized by authorities in every country. This is because there has never been any international agreement on the matter. In the past some scientists, believing that they had discovered a new vitamin, merely took the next letter in the alphabet for themselves and added another number to a series!

All this happened because the chemists working between 1930 and 1950 did not have the use of the advanced scientific instruments now available to identify chemical structures. The earlier workers would have extracted a mixture from a plant which they believed had vitamin-like properties, i.e. seemed essential for health. The mixture that they produced appeared to be quite different from other vitamins so they gave it a name, say vitamin U. Later researchers, using more modern methods, have found such substances were not vitamins but complex mixtures with an established vitamin as the principal component. Some of the items of the period are discredited as vitamins but it would be a brave person who said that the researchers were deliberately misleading people. They just did not have the equipment. Even today, with very up-to-date instruments, we cannot be sure that we have discovered every vitamin.

Great controversy rages over the difference between a natural vitamin and a synthetic one. In terms of defined chemical structure, there is no difference in most cases. However, things are not that simple. The term 'organic' is often used in this context but it is meaningless since all vitamins are organic – they all contain a basic carbon structure within their make-up. Carbon compounds are all defined chemically as organic whether they are made synthetically or from natural sources. All fresh foods will contain natural vitamins in minute quantities. Analysis of the food will break it down into all its components but the analysis will never be 100%, even with the most complex technological procedures available to the chemists. The analyst will find many of the items present but never achieve total breakdown and will therefore never be able to construct an identical food synthetically because of the lack of knowledge of all the natural components present.

The scientific nutritionists will not admit that the part of the food which has not been discovered on analysis could have any relevance to its nutritional value. The followers of the holistic health movement would disagree and say that the deficiency in knowledge of the whole structure is of vital importance and true natural vitamins contain elements which are not known to science but are all important to their function. It is a philosophical argument which is unlikely ever to be won. As scientific methods improve, they will get ever nearer to total analysis but never actually reach it and there will always be enough for the natural holistic people to cling on to.

Right may well be with the holistic movement because natural vitamins do appear to have extra properties when compared with synthetics. We define a natural vitamin as one occuring in its whole environment, whilst a synthetic is one solely prepared in the laboratory. A synthetic vitamin can be used as a booster to a natural vitamin in prepared supplements and there are even techniques for re-naturalizing being developed. This may make possible the wide production of natural vitamins under special conditions much as we can grow food efficiently using special techniques of soil fertilization. So you can see that there are degrees of naturalness, and makers of supplement concentrates like capsules and tablets have to compromise, but many are achieving high potencies of vitamins in surprisingly natural conditions for consumers.

□ *What are minerals?*

Chemistry recognizes two distinct groups of substances called organic and inorganic. Organic chemicals are all based upon the carbon atom whilst inorganic chemicals are derived from every other element. Minerals make up the major part of inorganic substances in nature, but in the body they are usually made into organic substances to form vital molecules – e.g. iron is bound into haemoglobin (a protein containing iron and carrying oxygen in the blood).

Minerals can only be taken into our bodies in food and none can be manufactured by the friendly organisms present in our intestines, as can some vitamins, or be prepared chemically by the body. For instance nicotinic acid (vitamin B3) can be prepared from the amino acid tryptophan. So from food we must obtain all the minerals we need in our diet. Not all minerals appear to be essential for health and some are poisonous, such as mercury and lead. Minerals occur throughout nature and inevitably in a mixed diet we will ingest both friendly and unfriendly ones. Of course, plants and other animals which provide our foods are equally harmed by the toxic minerals, so we ingest a minimum through eating healthy food because the harmful minerals have been filtered out for us. Unfortunately certain modern industrial processes use toxic minerals and pollution with these products and by-products has increased danger to human life from these minerals. Lead in petrol fumes has been a major concern recently and legislation in many countries bans the use of lead in petrol and diesel fuels. Many scientists believe that because of pollution by toxic minerals, our bodies need friendly nutrients in greater quantities than those required by our ancestors.

Recent advances in analytical chemistry have shown that some minerals, hitherto unsuspected of having an important role in nutrition, are present in our bodies. These minerals, like vanadium, nickel and molybdenum, are obtained in our food and deficiencies are thought to be rare.

Interest in these rarer minerals is likely to increase in the future. It is easier to detect the presence of minerals with modern analytical methods because their 'fingerprints' are all known to chemists. (New vitamins are different because we are looking for substances probably new to science and therefore without known chemical 'fingerprints'.)

Minerals are very stable chemically but they can be lost just as easily as vitamins through modern processing of foods. Fibrous parts of plants are rich in minerals but these play havoc with machinery in factories and shorten the working life of expensive grinders, cutters and blenders. They also make the end product less palatable – most people like smooth, creamy foods. Manufacturers process out the hard material which in fresh foods would be readily consumed, so the final processed food is deficient in minerals. Growing food on soils fertilized with synthetic chemicals can mean that the crops are deficient in trace elements which would be present if the soils were not so exhausted. Growing on areas where the crop is not naturally present can mean the same, because the new growing area may be deficient in trace elements normally found in the natural habitat.

Selenium is an element which is very important nutritionally and it has been shown that people who live in areas where the ground is low in selenium are more susceptible to cancer than those living on selenium rich soils. Continuing research into trace elements may well lead to further connections between certain diseases and particular concentrations of minerals in the soil. We have already had the example of cadmium, a dangerous mineral present to a high level in certain soils in the West Country, leading to health hazards for people eating vegetables grown on that soil.

Natural minerals are said to be better absorbed than synthetic ones. Synthetic minerals have many applications apart from nutritional ones and are very cheap. Food manufacturers often put back minerals in the synthetic form to compensate for the removal of the organic type in the processing. This happens with white bread, the iron and calcium being put back after the miller has removed the bran and the outer casing of the wheat. But what about the other minerals which might have been lost like molybdenum, selenium, nickel . . .?

When we talk about synthetic minerals, we mean sulphates, chlorides, selenites, molybdates etc. Using the more expensive amino acids, or gluconates or orotates, a closer approach to a natural mineral can be achieved. Such products are often called 'chelated'. As with vitamins, many manufacturers are endeavouring to get as close as possible to the mineral compounds actually found in foods when they make concentrates. Yeasts have been developed to yield true, naturally rich sources of chromium, selenium and molybdenum and these must represent the ultimate in processing for a truly natural mineral product. Soon other trace elements will be available in this form. Silica is one form of a mineral which has been available as a true natural concentrate for many years and manufacturers use an extract from a herb purified to be rich in natural silica.

☐ What are trace elements, amino acids and other nutrients?

Since this book is endeavouring to cover all the nutritional concentrates sold as products and ingredients in health stores, we have decided to look in some detail at all the items which are not strictly vitamins or minerals under this heading. We are not looking at compound formulas in this area, because they are too numerous. Furthermore, we are deliberately omitting most accepted herbs and herbal extracts, because although they are used in so-called 'diet supplements', the reason for the classification of the product under that heading is that the legal restrictions applying to herbal medicines can be avoided. This will explain the omission of details relating to items such as boldo, feverfew and yucca. Others, like alfalfa and spirulina, have been included and some of these can legitimately be called food concentrates because of specific high nutrient concentrations within their ingredient spectrum, e.g. vitamin B12 is rich in alfalfa, and vitamin F factor GLA (gamma linolenic acid) in spirulina. On the other hand, we are not aware of any essential nutrient or nutrients in feverfew, boldo or senna, all of which are found in diet supplements on health store shelves.

We shall, however, include some single chemically named ingredients which are not strictly nutrients, because their identity makes rational appraisal possible, e.g. DMSO.

Except for the amino acids, these items are all controversial as regards their nutritional benefits and classification. Nevertheless they must form an essential part of this book because consumers are using them and alternative practitioners are recommending them. Amino acids are all derived from food proteins and are used by the body to build its own protein. It is generally accepted that all food protein must be completely broken down to individual amino acids before absorption into the blood stream.

Some research has shown that compounds consisting of more than one amino acid can also be absorbed, and these peptide structures can be handled by the body for building its protein requirements. Insulin is a full protein structure and so cannot be absorbed in the gut and has to be used by injection. Drugs which mimic the effect of insulin obviously act by chemical blocking in the body and interfere with protein metabolism to the benefit of blood sugar levels, but there are side effects on other body processes.

Enzymes are protein structures but we consider those that act in the digestive tract may in themselves be nutrients because they are a component in food that if present could be utilized by the body for its metabolism without change.

Glandular nutrition is becoming increasingly popular in the USA and may provide some unique structures for use as nutrients. This is very controversial and whilst glandular extracts will be found as bases in some supplements, the use of single glands is a specialist area. Nucleic acids and proteins have a vast number of forms and often they are specific to particular body organs. It may be best to consider the glands as rich sources of special forms of these structures until more is known of the precise nature of their ingredients.

□*Destruction of vitamins and minerals*

Because they are quite complex chemical substances, many vitamins in foods are usually destroyed by processing. Cooking and storage even in a freezer will also have a deleterious effect. Maximizing one's natural vitamin intake can only be achieved by buying or growing fresh food and eating it as soon as possible. Even relatively short periods of storage in freezers can deplete some vitamin strengths by over 50%. The more stable vitamins like B2 or folic acid can still be lost because they will dissolve in cooking water. If this is not used to make gravies or sauces, then they will be lost in the discarded strainings. A water-soluble mineral like potassium will be lost in the same way.

Factory processing inevitably has an unfortunate effect on the vitamin and mineral contents of food. The removal of fibres, skins and other coarse material to prepare a palatable smooth end product inevitably leads to losses of nutrients. Manufacturers putting back a few cheap synthetics afterwards as a replacement present us with an inadequate answer. The use of synthetic additives like preservatives, colours and flavours probably adds to the negative nutritional value achieved by the extensive processing. The argument that many synthetic preservatives not only protect the quality of the food but may themselves be beneficial as some sort of life-extending drugs is humbug. The processing itself was an unnecessary expense and we should be concentrating on producing and distributing, efficiently, fresh wholesome foods, which of themselves would be quite life-extending enough.

Apart from the over-processing of foods which destroys practically all trace nutrients, there are other influences at work too. Light and exposure to air will destroy many vitamins. This point is well illustrated when your apple goes brown after being cut and left for a few minutes. The vitamin C is being broken down by the oxygen in the air. If the apple was dried very quickly for processing, then very little vitamin C would be lost, but what manufacturers do is to add a chemical, sulphur dioxide, to apples before drying and this prevents destruction of the vitamin C. Yet it means that the food will ultimately contain traces of undesirable sulphates. Sometimes nitrites are added to fresh food to prevent deterioration and these are potentially very harmful because they form nitroso compounds which are cancer causing.

Modern lifestyles and habits also destroy vitamins and distort the body's needs for particular nutrients. It is now accepted by many doctors that smoking is an important factor in causing cancer. More controversial is smoking's effect on vitamin and mineral balances in the body. Smokers will absorb minerals through their smoke, some may be useful, but tobacco contains toxic minerals like lead as well, so there may be problems. Smoking is generally considered as an anti-vitamin practice and some 25 mg of vitamin C is said to be needed by the body to cope with the effects of just one cigarette. So smokers need a great deal more vitamin C than non-smokers to ensure they have enough to do the normal metabolic tasks apart from compensating for cigarette smoking. Similar vitamin C needs will apply to cigar and pipe smokers. Other vitamins are also destroyed by smoking and any smokers should ensure that they take plenty of vitamins, probably in the form of a comprehensive supplement as well as extra vitamin C on a regular basis.

Alcohol is another anti-vitamin substance and it is vitamin B which is particularly affected. Alcohol is a concentrated food which is rapidly absorbed in the bloodstream and therefore puts a great demand on the body's resources for detoxification, using vitamins and minerals as part of the processes. A supplement which includes the B complex, vitamin C and the minerals calcium, magnesium, zinc and chromium is particularly recommended. The addition of the amino acid glutamine should not be overlooked since this plays an important part in nerve metabolism which may be adversely affected by alcohol. The purer the form of alcohol which is drunk, the more vitamins and minerals will be required. Gin, vodka and spirits in general are the most demanding, whilst beers and lagers, because of their lower alcohol content and natural vitamin B levels (they are more complete foods than spirits), will provide less of a nutritional problem. However, they may give rise to other effects such as allergies and stomach problems.

Pollution is a word we hear a great deal these days and in all its forms it is anti-nutrient. Chemical pesticides and fertilizers play havoc with nature's balance and provide our bodies with new problems in detoxification. Some pesticides like DDT and 245T have already been banned in many countries because of their toxicity. Others are becoming implicated in causing allergies. All mean extra burdens on our body's survival apparatus, which needs adequate supplies of micronutrients to counteract these enemies within. Food grown using pesticides will contain chemical residues of these for us to eat and a chemical fertilizer will probably have ensured that the food itself does not provide us with the exact spectrum or balance of nutrients of previous crops. The body faces two major problems, new poisons to dispose of safely and a new balance of nutrients to work with. Awareness of these problems must make us ensure that somehow we see that our bodies are provided with sufficient trace nutrients in balance, either by eating genuinely nutritious foods or by taking properly made natural supplement nutrient concentrates.

Drugs are another anti-nutrient group of substances. Doctors acknowledge that antibiotics not only destroy the micro-organisms (bacteria) which cause illnesses, but at the same time kill the flora (the natural friendly bacteria) of the intestine which produce some vitamins for the body's use. This is why after a course of antibiotics many doctors prescribe a multivitamin product to supply the vitamins usually produced by these friendly bacteria. After a few weeks of normal diet and health the flora should have re-established themselves. Drugs also provide the body with detoxification problems and this leads to more nutrients being needed to ensure that this processing can take place. Some drugs actually interfere directly with the natural nutrients. For instance, PABA is affected by the sulphonamides and it is more likely that the body processes utilizing that nutrient will be distorted, with perhaps serious long-term consequences. Some drugs are incompatible with certain foodstuffs, e.g. mono-amine oxidase inhibiting anti-depressants (nardil and eutonyl) with cheese and milk. These are also incompatible with the amino acid tryptophan. People on certain low protein diets will also be restricted on amino acids. So if you are taking prescribed drugs of any kind, you will at some time need a good nutrient supplement, but before altering your diet or taking one, you must discuss it with the doctor who has prescribed the medicine. Even everyday drugs like aspirin and paracetamol need detoxifying by the body and so demand micronutrients from the body's resources.

Tea and coffee are often considered anti-nutrients as well as soft drinks and colas. Caffeine and food additives contained in these products put a strain on the nutrient stores of your body.

So you can see that many aspects of modern living can have harmful consequences on your body's needs for micronutrients. Luckily as well as the modern processed foods and fast lifestyles, we have developed food concentrates which have an all-important part to play in overcoming the problems created, but many people might prefer to go back in time and practise the healthier aspects of our ancestors' lifestyles.

□*Dangers and overdosing with vitamins*

Since vitamins are in such small amounts in food, it is almost impossible for symptoms of excessive intake to occur using normal foods. Once extraction and purification have taken place, then new possibilities arise. Most scientists agree that the vast majority of vitamins have no practical toxic level. It would take vast energy and cost resources to ingest the sort of amounts which could be really dangerous.

Some vitamins do present potential hazards if not correctly used and it is appropriate to draw these to the reader's attention.

The vitamin causing most concern is vitamin D. It has been argued that this substance should be classified as a hormone rather than a vitamin because it is such a biologically active substance. From the vitamin section (page 96) you will see that it comes in several different forms, but all play the vital part in calcium metabolism involving bone formation. Rickets is a disease caused when malnutrition and lack of sunlight produce ill-formed brittle bones. It was very common in former times but adjustment of the national diet to include foods rich in vitamin D have seen the disease eradicated. However, taking too much vitamin D will produce softening of the bone structure, an equally dangerous situation. In most countries, including Britain, strict limits are placed on vitamin D levels in food and supplements and although these may be too cautious, we would not recommend anyone taking more than 5000 iu of vitamin D as a daily supplement except under a doctor's prescription for rickets.

Vitamin K is another oil-soluble vitamin which is dangerous because it has a potent effect on the blood clotting mechanism in the body. Too much will therefore cause greater clotting of the blood, with the risk of thrombosis. People taking medication to prevent excessive blood clotting, e.g. those who have suffered heart attacks or strokes, would obviously be at risk if they took an excess of vitamin K. You will not find supplements of this substance on its own generally available, but it is found in minute amounts in compound multivitamin and mineral products.

Vitamin A may be the most notorious of the dangerous

vitamins, largely because of the carrot-juice man story. Readers may recall the publicity in Britain caused when a man died because he had ingested vast quantities of carrot juice. The media blamed the vitamin A content but it was apparent that he was extracting the juice using solvents other than water and it was probably those that really caused the damage. As a result of the adverse publicity, legal pressures now force supplement product strength down to less than useful levels. (It would have been better to allow the higher concentrations to continue with perhaps an appropriate warning on the labels.) Vitamin A is stored in the liver and when these stores are full, the excess needs to be excreted from the body. The human body cannot quickly break down the vitamin A for excretion, so high blood levels can build up and cause several health problems including jaundice, hair loss, nervous problems. In order to suffer from these problems, most people would need to take some 50,000 to 100,000 iu of vitamin A daily for several months on its own. All the reports of toxicity of vitamin A appear to refer to overdoses of the vitamin on its own or in vast excess. When it is used in conjunction with a multiplicity of other vitamins and minerals in a more balanced supplement, there seem to be no ill effects. Indeed, we know of one practitioner who has used very high doses of vitamin A in conjunction with a vitamin nutrition plan in the long-term treatment of eye health without any problems at all. Dr Stanley Evans, a practising ophthalmic nutritionist, has published his nutritional plans in several books. See *Nutrition in Eye Health and Disease* (Roberts Publications, London, 1983).)

The primary cause of the problem arising with vitamin A has been newspaper reports making out-of-context claims that vitamin A cures cancer. People then react by going out and taking vast amounts of the vitamin without reading that vitamins, like foods, should be taken as a balance. Would you just live on potatoes? Even water in excess can kill! Vitamin A is as important to health as vitamin C. Perhaps the best supplemental form to take it in is beta-carotene, the water-soluble form, but the problem here is that even a relatively low dose supplement will produce a yellowing of the skin which is unacceptable to many people. Beta carotene is certainly classified as non-toxic. Its water solubility enables it to be excreted easily by the body, as long as really excessive amounts are not taken.

In the 1980s some controversy arose about vitamin B6. This substance has been widely recommended for menstrual problems and especially for women on the pill. Unfortunately B6 alone does not help everyone, so some women have taken much more than recommended and in isolation from other nutrients. As a result, imbalances arise. Again we blame the media who give edited versions of scientific papers without emphasizing the holistic ideas of the nutritional approaches to health care.

Vitamin B12 and folic acid are restricted in nutritional use as supplements but not because of toxicity. They interfere with certain diagnostic tests used by doctors to detect serious disease like pernicious anaemia. We believe that it would be better to include a routine question to patients who are to take the tests. It would ask them if they took vitamin supplements regularly and particularly mention B12 and folic acid. The problem is that doctors seldom acknowledge any intelligence in their patients. This approach would appear to be more sensible than depriving the general population of effective supplemental levels of these two vital nutrients. In other countries, more enlightened approaches apply and the supplements with relatively high vitamin B12 and folic acid concentrations are well known.

It is important for these two substances that one should not be taken in complete isolation from the other. This is where the basic nutritional supplement of any regime is so vital.

Certain individuals may show sensitivity to excessive amounts of the vitamins and this is why it is wise not to take highly concentrated supplements without reliable advice. Doses exceeding RDA by a factor of more than 10 could be generally considered as the maximum to use without such advice.

People have found increased laxative effects with some vitamins in large doses, especially vitamin C and a number of the B group including pantothenic acid. If large doses in excess of the RDA are recommended to you, it is sensible to build up to these levels gradually over a 7 to 14 day period to enable your body to accustom itself to the extra nutrient.

We have covered the major items regarding overdosing with vitamins and other nutrients. While doubtless there will be more in the future, we are certain they will arise because of a lack of understanding of the wholeness necessary in the approach to nutritional treatments. We admit that this is complex and not easy for scientific assessment, but that should not preclude their use, particularly when drug treatments can be so hazardous.

Because the body is able to excrete excess of most vitamins through natural processes, overdosing is rare. See information on individual vitamins and minerals in the appropriate section of this book.

■5 Nutrients in pill and capsule form

□ Vitamins and nutrients in 'pills'

Magazines and newspapers frequently carry articles on vitamin pills (tablets and capsules) and vastly different views are expressed. The public is definitely confused by the experts but personal experience seems to be so good that sales increase well above expectations every year despite the huge vested interests (the food industry and the medical profession) ranged against them. Many health stores have vast ranges of supplements on offer, some supermarkets are even stocking own brand copies of the popular advertised products. Chain store chemists and health stores have own brands or predominantly stock brands which either offer them huge discounts or are made by companies within the group.

The involvement of big business means that many products on offer to the public lack the vital components of wholeness. This is because the fundamental concepts behind natural vitamins tend to become lost in the profit jungle. There is nothing the consumer can do about this apart from withdrawing his custom from products which emanate from these sources. Don't forget these products serve the purpose of at least stimulating interest in nutrition because the advertising money invested in them is very large. Unfortunately they do not give the really satisfactory results associated with the naturally-based products. We hope consumers will come to realize that a vitamin supplement needs a basic formula different from a simple drug like aspirin or paracetamol.

Companies involved in capsule and tablet manufacture (genuine pills are virtually non-existent these days – we only use the term because it is widely understood colloquially) depend for most of their income on drugs. They employ experts in that particular area of formulation.

When a manufacturing chemist makes paracetamol tablets he uses the chemically pure ingredients he was taught about in col-

lege or has been sold by the fine chemicals industry. Pure paracetamol is a powder and requires several additives to be used
before it can be made into a tablet. A 500 mg tablet of paracetamol
will probably weigh about 700 mg and the other 200 mg will
consist of various fillers and binders, for example modified
starches, synthetic gums like polyvinylpyrrolfidone, lubricants
like mineral oil and chemical preservatives. Exact formulas will
vary between manufacturers and this is why there is controversy
about bio-availability of the active ingredients. Do you remember
the advertisement that said 'nothing acts faster'? That is because
the manufacturers considered that their product broke down in
the stomach quicker for rapid absorption and use of the active
constituents by the body, because the additives they had used gave
the preparation those properties.

A capsule manufacturer needs additives to bulk up the product
to fit the gelatin shell required. In turn the shell is prepared from
ingredients apart from gelatin including glycerin, chemical
plasticizers and preservatives. In addition soft gelatin capsules are
dried using special chemical solvents, and slight residues of these
remain at the end of the process in minute amounts.

If the tablet or capsule is coloured, it usually means that
synthetic dyes have been used, and for flavours similar criteria
would apply. Particularly reprehensible is the widespread use of
sugar in tablets, a practice condemned by many doctors because it
can play havoc with teeth, especially in chewable products and
children's medicines. Tablets are often coated and this may be
with either sugar or protein these days. Another form of tablet
coating is called enteric and it is used for both capsules and
tablets. It protects ingredients from attack by the stomach juices
and allows the tablet or capsule to pass beyond the stomach before
releasing its contents. Sometimes these coatings do not work
effectively and the product passes right through your digestive
tract. At other times it may break up in the colon (large intestine)
where the ingredients cannot be effectively absorbed and this may
cause local irritation of the gut lining, which may be dangerous.
Coating a tablet can make it as elegant looking as a capsule but it
will need additives to achieve the elegance necessary for
pharmaceutical purposes. Appearance and presentation are
essential so that the pharmacist can prove to the doctor what a
professional he is. It also enables companies to brand their products by appearance as well as name – an all important point in
the fight about generic substitution. The patients are familiar
with a blue slimming tablet with a trade mark on it, they will
certainly complain and probably get less satisfaction from a plain
unmarked white tablet, despite the active ingredients being
identical.

Recently a drug company was successful in a legal case which gave it the proprietary rights in a particular combination of mixed colours for capsule shells for a particular ingredient. Manufacturers who wanted to compete with them had to put that same drug material in a different combination of colours. As a result the patients would certainly be confused if the doctors did not stick with the original proprietary brand.

These examples illustrate what a jungle confronts the manufacturer of natural vitamins. Most makers who are familiar with drugs will approach vitamin formulas in the traditional way. But vitamins are foods not drugs. Most chemists would reply that they are all just chemicals to be made acceptable for human consumption. We believe that there is a difference between drugs and vitamins. Drugs are foreign to the body while vitamins are not. It is right to package or formulate vitamins and minerals in as near a natural environment as possible so as to give the body fewer problems to solve when they are taken. Vitamins should be made as foods and not as if they were drugs, and a different approach to making the tablets and capsules is essential.

Analysis of ingredients is becoming more and more important. The complex natural formulations for a vitamin product mean problems for the analytical chemist when he comes to do his job. A simple formula with known chemical additives makes the work of the analyst easy. Should we sacrifice the ideals of a natural vitamin product on the altar of the chemical analyst? We think not. Authorities do not agree and there are likely to be problems in the future for natural vitamins because of the sheer obstinacy of the bureaucrats even to consider our philosophy. They will want total analysis as a first priority because they are technologically brainwashed and believe in the infallibility of scientific method.

If you are looking for a *natural* vitamin supplement, look out for the following points:

1 All ingredients should be clearly stated on the label, including non-actives, i.e. additives used.

2 Chemical additives listed should have details so that you can tell what chemical has been used at a glance. E numbers are not sufficient – who carries an E number code book to the health food shop or chemist?

3 If a product is brightly coloured or bi-coloured (some capsules are half one colour and half another) it won't be very natural.

4 Whiteness seldom equates with naturalness but may equate with the term 'nature identical'.

5 Chewability is a warning sign. Inositol, the B vitamin, is very pleasant to chew but we have never seen it used as a base in chewable tablets (see later for more details, p. 64).

6 Look at the bases used: if herbs and proteins are included this is a plus sign, but if no declaration about freedom from additives is present be cautious.

7 Freedom from preservatives is a good indicator but beware of this claim if it is not also aligned to 'additive free' because there are lots of permitted chemical additives besides preservatives.

8 See if natural preservatives are used. Vitamins C and E act as such in both capsules and tablets quite satisfactorily.

9 Letters after ingredients like BP or USP, whilst indicating the use of processed substances, may be forced upon manufacturers by legal authorities' requirements. They certainly equate with the term 'nature identical'.

10 Sugar comes in many forms of description and mention of any of the following means that substantial amounts of refined sugar or sucrose may be present in the tablets:

> sucrose
> molasses or dried molasses
> turbinados sugar
> saccharinose
> honey or dried honey
> cane sugar
> natural cane sugar
> root sugar
> beet sugar
> raw sugar
> icing sugar
> fruit sugar (probably a mixture of sucrose and fructose
> where fructose is less than 1% of the total)

11 Sweeteners present – sorbitol, mannitol, xylitol, saccharin, aspartame.

You will find two kinds of basic formulated vitamin supplements –tablets and capsules. Most capsules are a soft, smooth ovoid (oval) totally sealed package of oily liquid; a few are what are called hard shelled, usually filled with dry powder and coming in two halves with a base and a cap, which can be parted, sometimes with difficulty, to empty out the contents. Tablets are hard and come in many shapes, predominantly round but increasingly ovoid for easy swallowing. Tablets are usually plain, just sealed or protein coated. Rarely are they sugar coated although this is still a popular presentation, especially in the underdeveloped world where elegance is important for an imported product from the USA or Europe. Tablets are all prepared by compressing dry powders. Hard gelatin capsules, the sort with the tops and the bottoms, are prepared like tablets and need similar types of for-mulation to achieve their ends economically.

The hard gelatin capsule would be much better, but again could not satisfy vegetarian requirements and is very costly be-cause two processes have to be carried out quite separately – the preparation of the shell and then its filling. A soft capsule is made in one operation.

Hard capsules may be coloured and probably contain additives even when clear. Small-scale hand production of filled hard gelatin capsules can be done without additives but commercially production can only be achieved by use of additives to ensure that the mixtures flow on the machine and into the shells consistently.

Soft gelatin capsules are the most elegant and consistent pre-sentation for drugs and vitamins. Considerable technology is re-quired to achieve this and processing is expensive. The products are not suitable for vegetarians or vegans because gelatin only comes from animal sources. Whether a capsule could ever be described as a 'natural' product is certainly open to argument. One of the major disadvantages of the soft capsule is not its cost but the fact that it must have an oily inside. If it did not, the gelatin shell would liquefy. This means that the body has to get the ingredients through an oil and this seems a most unnatural en-vironment for the water-soluble vitamins like C and B. Its pro-perties as a stable and elegant product mean that the capsule will be with us for many years but should obviously not be the first choice for a natural non-oily vitamin or mineral product.

After the natural food, a freeze-dried powder of it is probably the most nutritious form. In order to prepare tablets and capsules, powders will be needed and obviously those powders should be made as carefully as possible to ensure potency of nutrients over a long period. A powder forming a base for a natural food supplement concentrate should be prepared in ideal conditions and meet a standard specification of essential nutrients. This aim is seldom achievable and manufacturers 'adjust' their powders to ensure the potency. A good example of a vitamin powder is acerola berry powder. This comes from Puerto Rico and contains a guaranteed level of vitamin C. This is not achieved using just acerola berries but by adding processed vitamin C to acerola powder. The natural dried powder may only yield about 2% of vitamin C, but with the addition of processed vitamin C, this will be increased to 25%. It would be wrong to call this 100% natural vitamin C as many manufacturers do, but it may be preferable to standard processed C of 99% purity used by drug manufacturers and the makers of supermarket vitamins.

Manufacturers of natural vitamins always incorporate some of nature's source of the vitamin in their products to ensure that the full spectrum of nutrients is present in the final product. The exception to this would be when a product is required for people who are sensitive to food factors and need only the pure ingredients to be present in the product. Bioflavonoid factors known as vitamin P are usually incorporated in natural vitamin C products together with acerola and rose hip powders. In vitamin A products you should find some beta-carotene and with many B vitamins yeast or whole cereal bases are used to provide nature's filler factors.

Calcium supplements in chemist shops are usually derived from calcium lactate but in herbal stores you will find bonemeal and dolomite as the calcium sources. Chelates (compounds where minerals are bound organically) like proteinates and orotates are the normal sources of minerals in natural health products, but in chemist shops you will find sulphates and chlorides (inorganic) used. If sulphates have to be used in supplements, responsible manufacturers will ensure protein and amino acid factors are in the formula to assist natural chelation to help absorption by the body.

The tablet is certainly the usual form of food supplement concentrate found in the world. Largely for economic reasons the tablet is the most widely found form of drug preparation and therefore this has lead to its adoption by natural vitamin makers. The tablet does provide certain advantages over soft capsules and these advantages are not to be lightly discredited. Tablets can be made which come very close to providing the body with very food-like properties. The ingredients are in dry powder form and so need only a minimum of processing from the fresh product to render it fit for tabletting. If pure forms of vitamins are needed to yield high potencies, then it is simple to treat them with the natural gums that bind them into the tablet so that they are yielded steadily to the body (sustained release) as if in a natural food – the body working in its normal way to obtain the vital nutrient. Remember a soft capsule is oil based and this is not a 'natural' environment for most nutrients. Many powders are absorbent and can be used to carry oily vitamins in very finely divided form so that the body gets these nutrients as it would in foods as minute particles. Oily vitamins are found in minute fatty particles in food, not in large dollops as they are when given in capsule form. Sometimes capsule makers emulsify the oil with pectin or other fibre, but still the overall environment is oil. We believe that vitamin E, one of the oily vitamins, is best taken as a tablet. A capsule may be more potent and more expensive, but when swallowed it will not give the nutritional value promised. So much of the oil may pass through the body unused because natural emulsification will not be satisfactorily achieved.

Whilst the plain, sustained release and protein film coated tablets are potentially the most natural form of supplement obtainable, please check labels even of these products carefully.

There are two forms of tablet of which you must be extremely wary: these are the *sugar coated* and the *chewable*. Both would almost certainly contain refined sugar (sucrose) in one form or another.

We have found chewable tablets among the most misleadingly labelled products on health food store shelves. Most of the bestselling lines are chewable tablets, especially vitamin C, but manufacturers have gone to great lengths to deceive consumers. In this they have been aided by the makers of so-called 'sugarless' bases for chewable tablets. Two of the notorious bases are powdered honey and powdered molasses. They are both brown in colour and they smell of the products mentioned, yet they are in fact almost pure sucrose. They are made by dissolving a little molasses or a little honey in concentrated sugar syrup and then performing a process called spray-drying on the solution. The result is the two powders which are then (innocently?) used by tabletters to produce the gorgeous-tasting goodies that children and even adults love. In the USA some ten chewable vitamin C products were tested and nine had over 50% of sugar present yet all were labelled sugar-free. The remaining one had just under 50% sugar.

□ *Which multivitamin should I take?*

Most people who use vitamins and minerals do not just take single concentrates but use a basic supplement containing a large spectrum of vitamins and minerals. We have all heard the slogans and jingles for the popular brands which usually provide just the recommended daily allowance values of the recognized vitamins. Sometimes these brands actually yield only three or four vitamins in total.

Multinutrient products are a rich source of variety with some formulas embracing almost 100 ingredients. References to 'plus' and 'extra potency' 'super strength', must leave the average consumer baffled. Our advice is to stick to a brand which provides a wide spectrum of nutrients, suits you and makes believable claims in advertising. The addition of one magic new ingredient is unlikely to be worth the extra cost. Worthwhile amounts of specific nutrients like vitamin E, C, or tonics like ginseng will only generally be obtained by the use of a single concentrate of that particular item.

There are some nutrient concentrate products of a special kind which contain just a few ingredients in specific balances. These are sometimes of real help, but care is needed in distinguishing the properly researched product from a gimmicky mixture made to cash in on the back of an original product.

So use your multinutrient supplement as a base and build on it according to your needs and don't forget the natural style of diet, which is more important than anything else.

■6   Vitamins

■Vitamin A

Retinol, vitamin A1, also vitamin A2 a close chemical relative of retinol called dehydroretinol. Neo vitamin A, a natural form of vitamin A and more stable than retinol. Pro vitamin A (see Beta-carotene, page 69).

□*Fat-soluble*

□*Natural sources*   Animal liver, particularly fish oils, e.g. cod liver and halibut liver. (Polar bear liver is very rich in vitamin A and can be toxic if eaten to excess.) Plants do not contain retinol but many are rich in carotenoids including beta-carotene, which is converted to vitamin A by the liver. For beta-carotene, see page 69.

□*Synthetic forms*   To prepare concentrates, vitamin A can be synthesized commercially by many routes including using natural starting materials such as beta-carotene. It is stabilized by conversion to an ester form using organic acids such as acetic for retinol acetate or palmitic for retinol palmitate.

□*Main functions in the body*   Protection from infection; good for eye health – without adequate vitamin A vision is impaired; skin tissue also needs it to keep its elasticity. It has anti-cancer properties but must not be taken to excess – 7,500 iu (international unit) daily is adequate for healthy people.

□*Main deficiency symptoms*   Night blindness, itching and burning eyes, dry hair and rough skin.

□*Main co-vitamins*   Vitamin D with which it occurs in fish oils, vitamin C where there is a combined protective effect against infections, and this helps overcome toxic effects of too much vitamin A.

□*Overdosing and toxicity*   Vitamin A is stored in the liver and if large doses (50,000 – 100,000 iu daily) are taken for a prolonged period, the liver cannot store the vitamin A and it builds up in the body to give unpleasant side-effects which include headaches, hair loss, nausea, drowsiness and weight loss.

Nutritional courses with doses of 25,000 iu or more should be taken at intervals of 3 weeks on a daily basis and then resting for 3–4 weeks before another course. This enables the stored vitamin A to be used and will prevent saturation. Pro vitamin A (beta-carotene) does not create this problem.

□*Stability*　Vitamin A is destroyed by air and sunlight, the speed of destruction depending on both its chemical constitution and the form of preparation or food in which it is situated. Freezing of fish will deplete its natural vitamin A content and so will cooking.

□*Product types and best buys*　Capsules are the most stable pharmaceutical form of retinol. Tablets, powders and suspensions if properly made are stable but should be used within 3 months of opening the container. Tablets with beta-carotene (Pro vitamin A) yielding about 50% source of vitamin A are probably the best buy for supplementary insurance purposes.

□*RDA (Recommended Daily Amount) and units*　Retinol sets the basic standard for all vitamin A products. A term widely used is the retinol equivalent and to complicate matters this is quite different from the long established international unit (iu). A retinol equivalent of vitamin A activity is equal to that of one mcg of pure retinol, and one mcg of retinol yields 3.33 iu of vitamin A. In the UK, the RDA for adult males is 750 mcg retinol or 2,500 iu, whereas in the USA it is 1,500 retinol equivalents or 5000 iu, with a recommendation that half be from retinol itself and the remainder from beta-carotene. Children require less, depending on age, and women during pregnancy and lactation more. In the USA, women have a RDA of 4000 iu.

□*Research and bibliography*　Book: *The Vitamins*, vol. 1, W. H. Sebrell and R. S. Harris (Academic Press, New York, 2nd Edition, 1967).

Retinol (Vitamin A) content of foods
in mcg per 100 g

* *best sources*

bread/flours/grains	0
vegetables/fruit/nuts	0
vegetable oils	0

most fish	*trace*
bacon	*trace*
beef	*trace*
lamb	*trace*
pork	*trace*
chicken	*trace*
* fried calf liver	17,400
* fried chicken liver	11,000
* fried lamb's liver	20,600
* stewed ox liver	20,100
* stewed pig's liver	9,200
* cod liver oil	18,000
butter	750
margarine	900
egg	140
canned salmon	90
fried cod's roe	150
raw oysters	75
whole milk	26 – 35
dried skimmed milk	*trace*
single cream	145 – 200
double cream	330 – 450
Cheddar cheese	310
Stilton	370
cottage cheese	32
natural yoghurt (unfortified)	8
shortbread	230
sponge cake (with fat)	300
mince pies	90
shortcrust pastry	160

The figures for milk vary according to season, with milk produced in winter containing less retinol than that produced in summer. Figures for cream also reflect the same trend. Liver is by far the best source of retinol, but as many people do not like it, margarine and butter are more likely to be important sources of this vitamin in the average diet. High fat cheeses such as Cheddar contain more retinol than the low fat varieties such as cottage cheese.

Here is a recipe for a high retinol food that will make eight portions. It can be stored in the fridge for two or three days if covered tightly.

Chicken liver pâté

Ingredients 1 lb (500 g) chicken livers (frozen or fresh), 1 small onion, 2 tablespoons sunflower oil, 1 clove garlic, 2 pinches mixed herbs, black pepper, 2 teaspoons sherry or port, 1 tablespoon milk or single cream, 1 tablespoon soy sauce.

Method Pick over the livers, remove and discard any stringy or yellow pieces. Wash and dry on kitchen paper. Chop into smallish pieces. Peel and finely chop the onion. Put the oil into a frying pan and gently fry the onion for about 4 to 5 minutes but don't let it brown. Add the garlic, peeled and put through a garlic crusher. Put in the herbs, chopped chicken livers and 2 or 3 grinds black pepper. Use a wooden spoon to stir/fry, slightly increasing the heat. Continue for about 5 minutes by which time the livers should be crumbly and cooked. Allow to cool a little and then put into a blender with the alcohol, milk or cream and soy sauce. Blend to a smooth paste. If it turns out rather thin, put back into the pan and heat to make a stiffer paste. Spoon into small dishes and allow to cool. Serve chilled from the fridge with hot, wholewheat toast.

(A food processor can be used instead of a blender for this recipe.)

■Beta-carotene and the carotenes (pro vitamin A)

The water-soluble forms of vitamin A, alpha and gamma carotenes, also occur naturally but are not so readily converted to vitamin A by the body.

□*Natural sources* Green vegetables, carrots – but not fish oils.

□*Commercial forms used for supplements* It can be made synthetically, and most is derived using fermentation processes. Extraction from plants is very expensive. Commercial forms are usually beadlets which give prolonged stability. It is used as a colouring agent in foods. E 160 (a) is its E number.

□*Main functions* See Vitamin A, page 66. It is used as a sunscreen.

□*Main deficiency symptoms* See Vitamin A.

□*Co-vitamins* See Vitamin A.

□*Stability* Pure beta-carotene absorbs oxygen from the air and loses potency as a result. The beadlets of commerce are very stable for use in supplements.

□*Overdosing and toxicity*   Much safer than vitamin A as the body can excrete excess quite easily because of this vitamin's water solubility. Large doses, over 10,000 iu daily, will produce yellow colouring of the skin which is unacceptable to many people.

□*RDA*   See Vitamin A. 1 iu of vitamin A activity is found in approximately 0.6 mcg of beta-carotene. Alpha-carotene is less active, 1.2 mcg being needed for 1 iu of vitamin A.

Carotene (Vitamin A, alpha/beta/gamma carotenes) content of foods
in mcg per 100 g

* *best sources*

breads/flours/grains	0
nuts	0
shortbread	140
fresh milk	26 – 35
dried, skimmed milk	*trace*
butter	470
margarine	0
single cream	70 – 125
double cream	160 – 280
Cheddar cheese	250
Parmesan	195
cottage cheese	18
natural yoghurt	5
eggs	*trace*
meat	*trace*
fried calf liver	100
fried lamb's liver	60
stewed ox liver	1540
stewed pig's liver	0
boiled asparagus	250
boiled French beans	400
boiled runner beans	400
boiled broad beans	250
* broccoli tops boiled	2500
boiled Brussels sprouts	400
raw white cabbage	0
raw red cabbage	*trace*
* raw or cooked old carrots	12000

* raw or cooked young carrots	6000
* raw endive	2000
lettuce	1000
mushrooms	0
mustard and cress	500
onions	0
raw parsley	7000
peas	300
raw or cooked green peppers	200
potatoes	*trace*
* boiled spinach	6000
* boiled spring greens	4000
tomatoes	600
* boiled turnip tops	6000
* watercress	3000
fresh apricots	1500
* dried apricots	3600
bananas	200
dates	50
fresh figs	500
grapes	*trace*
raw mangoes	1200
* raw Cantaloupe melon	2000
yellow Honeydew melon	100
watermelon	20
fresh peaches	500
raw dried peaches	2000
raw prunes	1000
tomato purée	2860
tomato sauce	1230

Highly coloured foods are the best sources. Note the type of melon with the highest level of carotene is one with orange flesh. In dried fruits the levels of this vitamin are higher than in the fresh. Cooking does not necessarily mean loss of carotene.

■Vitamin B1/thiamin, aneurine

Usual label designation is thiamin hydrochloride or thiamin mononitrate.

□*Water-soluble.*

□*Natural sources* Whole grain, cereals, brewer's yeast, wheat germ, meats. Has a very characteristic clingy smell often associated with breweries and bakeries.

71

□*Commercial forms for use in supplements* Several methods of synthesis are available, and all commercial products are prepared using the synthetic hydrochloride or mononitrate. Isolation and extraction from natural sources is not commercially viable.

□*Main functions* In the metabolism of carbohydrates. It forms part of the enzyme cocarboxylase which is essential in the Krebs cycle for conversion of carbohydrate to energy. It helps overcome neuritis and one of its names, aneurine, derived from its benefit to nerves.

□*Main deficiency symptoms* Extreme deficiency causes the disease beriberi. Other effects include fatigue, anorexia, stomach and digestion disturbances, as well as nervousness and irritability.

□*Main co-factors* Other members of the B complex, especially vitamin B2, folic acid and nicotinic acid.

□*Overdosing and toxicity* There is no known toxic level, but taking more than 500 mg daily on a regular basis is unnecessary. As a supplement it is usually taken as part of a general B complex, in amounts of 1 to 10 mg daily.

□*Stability* Freezing and cooking will cause losses if the water is discarded at any stage. Otherwise very stable and properly made supplement concentrates will keep their potency for many years even in less than ideal conditions.

□*RDA and units* Before the days of chemical assay, a unit of activity for this vitamin was established. This was subsequently found to be 33 iu per mg thiamin. Thiamin is almost always declared on labels as the hydrochloride or mononitrate, and the RDA is about 1 to 1.5 mg daily, with more for the elderly (2 mg) and less for very young children (0.5 mg). An insurance supplement of 5 mg daily is enough for most people, but for extra security many people take more and there is no toxicity problem. B1 should always be adequately balanced with B2 and nicotinic acid.

□*Research and bibliography* American New York Academy of Science, 378, *Thiamine: 20 years of progress*, H. Z. Sable and C. J. Grubier (1982).

Thiamin (Vitamin B 1) content of foods

in mg per 100 g

* *best sources*

wheat germ	1.45
wheat bran	0.89

raw oatmeal	0.50
low fat soya flour	0.90
* bread with wheat germ	0.52
All-Bran	0.75
* Special K	1.7
* Weetabix	1.0
dried skimmed milk	0.42
raw egg yolk	0.30
average lean bacon	0.65
* average lean pork	0.89
heart	0.45
fried lamb's kidney	0.56
* ham	0.52
fried cod's roe	1.3
fresh, boiled peas	0.25
almonds	0.24
* brazils	1.00
* fresh peanuts	0.90
meat extract spread	3.1
dried yeast	2.33
brewer's yeast	15.6

Fats, oils, beef, lamb, chicken, fish, most vegetables and fruit are all poor sources of this vitamin. It is added to some breakfast cereals during manufacture, which accounts for their contribution to thiamin in the diet. As they can be eaten in quite large amounts they are a valuable source. By making your own bread and adding wheat germ as an extra, as well as soya flour (low fat), the thiamin value of your daily bread can be increased. Although brewer's yeast looks like an extra good source, bear in mind that figure is for 100 g (approximately 4 oz), which happens to be quite a large number of tablets (about 330 × 300 mg tablets).

■Vitamin B2/riboflavin, lactoflavin, also called vitamin G

Food additive E 101.
Water-soluble (slightly), but more soluble in body fluids.

□*Natural sources* Yeast, milk, eggs, green vegetables, liver, kidney. Riboflavin is found in cells throughout the animal and plant kingdoms.

□*Synthetic forms* Riboflavin phosphate sodium is a special synthetic form used for preparing injections and liquid pharmaceutical preparations. There are several synthetic methods for riboflavin's preparation, but natural bacterial fermentation processes are the most widely used.

□*Main functions* It is only found as riboflavin in the retina of the eye, otherwise it is combined in complex molecules in body cells. In the combined form it plays a vital part in enzyme systems for oxidative and respiration processes. It is especially associated with eye and skin health.

□*Main deficiency symptoms* Mouth sores, itching eyes, eye fatigue, even blindness and cataracts. Red sore tongue, burning feet, oily skin, nasal and anal sores.

□*Main co-factors* Phosphorus, needed to ensure utilization of other B group vitamins, especially B1 and B6.

□*Overdosing and toxicity* No known toxic level, but in excess it will yield a bright yellow colour to the urine. This indicates that the body has sufficient of the vitamin for its needs. As a supplement, more than an equivalent amount to that of vitamin B1 is seldom needed. Most nutritionists prefer B1 and B2 to be equal in potency in a compound supplement, but this is not a universal view.

□*Stability* Very stable, but could be lost if green vegetables are overcooked and the water discarded. Supplements will have a long shelf life.

□*RDA* 1.3 to 1.8 mg, but increases during pregnancy and breastfeeding to over 2 mg. As a nutritional insurance 5 mg daily may be used as a supplement form. If more, then it is preferable to balance it with other B group vitamins, especially B1 and B3.

Riboflavin (Vitamin B2) content of foods

in mg per 100 g

* *best sources*

wheat germ	0.61
low fat soya flour	0.36
* cornflakes	1.6
* Rice Krispies	1.7
* Special K	1.9
* Weetabix	1.5
fresh milk	0.19
dried, skimmed milk	1.6

Camembert type cheese	0.60
Parmesan	0.50
Cheddar	0.50
yoghurt	0.26
boiled egg, raw egg	0.45
poached egg	0.38
lean, grilled rumpsteak	0.40
lean roast duck	0.47
roast grouse	0.54
roast sheep's heart	1.5
stewed ox heart	1.1
* kidney	2.3
* fried calf's liver	4.2
* fried chicken liver	3.3
* fried lamb's liver	3.1
* stewed ox heart	3.6
* stewed pig's liver	3.1
fried cod's roe	0.9
milk chocolate	0.23
* almonds	0.92
chestnuts	0.22
dried yeast	4.0

Fortified breakfast cereals and liver are the best sources of this vitamin in the diet. There are some losses on cooking, as the figures for raw egg and poached egg show. Note the boiled egg, being neatly sealed in the shell, has the same as the raw egg for vitamin value. Vegetarians can acquire most of their riboflavin from eggs, cheese and almonds.

■ Vitamin B3 – niacin or nicotinic acid

Niacinamide or nicotinamide (also known as vitamin PP) is also a substance generally accepted as B3. Pantothenic acid has also been referred to as B3, but we prefer to classify this substance as B5.

□*Water-soluble* Niacin (nicotinic acid) more soluble than nicotinamide.

□*Natural sources* Eggs, whole grains, meat, milk, organ meats, nuts, seafood, poultry, liver, yeast, rice polishings.

□*Commercial forms for supplements* Nicotinamide is a synthetic compound derived chemically from nicotinic acid. Niacin (nicotinic acid) is converted into nicotinamide in the body.

Niacin is only commercially available in the synthetic form derived from nicotine or pyridine.

□*Main functions*   Antipellagra substance (pellagra is the classic deficiency disease, with appetite loss, fatigue, diarrhoea, marked skin eruptions and mental disturbance). Niacin is converted to the nicotinamide form in the body, so by using nicotinamide instead of niacin you do not impair nutrition. Vitamin B3 has been particularly used to help schizophrenia and other mental conditions in high doses. It lowers LDL and VLDL levels in the blood, which makes it useful as an aid to heart disease, but the doses required are fairly high – 3 g daily is quoted. (LDL is Low Density Lipoprotein, and VLDL is Very Low Density Lipoprotein. These are substances in the blood which have significantly higher concentrations in people who are susceptible to heart attacks.)

□*Main deficiency symptoms*   Pellagra.

□*Co-vitamins*   B1, B2, B6 (which helps produce B3 with amino acid tryptophan), phosphorus.

□*Overdosing and toxicity*   Nicotinic acid should not be given to patients with peptic ulcers because of its vasodilator effects. It may potentiate (make worse) health problems such as skin rashes and nausea. Nicotinic acid produces vasodilation, which leads to severe flushing of the skin. This flushing can occur with fairly small doses, e.g. 10 mg and is very marked when 100 mg or greater doses are used. The flushing soon passes off, but people should be warned of this effect, which can be quite alarming when unexpected.

□*Stability*   Very stable in supplements.

□*RDA*   15 to 20 mg, but could be much more as a nutritional insurance. 100 mg would not be excessive if taken as nicotinamide.

□*Bibliography*   *The Vitamins*, vol. 3, W. H. Sebrell & R. S. Harris (Academic Press, New York, 1954), pp. 596, 598.

■Vitamin B4/Adenine

□*Natural sources*   Occurs naturally in nucleic acids RNA and DNA and is found throughout animal and plant tissues, usually in association with vitamin B3.

May be prepared synthetically. It is not an officially recognized vitamin. It is needed to build nucleic acids in the body and also takes part in enzyme systems.

■Vitamin B5

Pantothenic acid, calcium D-pantothenate. Niacin and niacinamide are sometimes referred to as B5, but we prefer to classify these as B3.

□*Water-soluble*

□*Natural sources* Dates, cereals, brewer's yeast, eggs, mushrooms, liver, legumes, green vegetables, peanuts, milk, royal jelly, bran and molasses.

□*Commercial form for supplements* All commercial forms of pantothenic acid are made synthetically using beta alanine (an amino acid). Pantothenic acid is an oily substance which is not very stable, so the calcium pantothenate form is used to prepare supplements. Only the D form is nutritionally useful.

□*Main functions* As a component of coenzyme A in the Krebs energy cycle. It plays an important part in the formation of the cortico-steroid hormones in the adrenal gland and is depleted in stressful conditions. Aids the immune system generally.

□*Main deficiency symptoms* Fatigue, poor hair condition, adrenal exhaustion, sleep disturbance, stomach disorder. Barton Wright, an English bio-chemist, was convinced that arthritis was caused by long term deficiency.

□*Co-vitamins* B6, B12, biotin and folic acid.

□*Stability* Pantothenic acid is unstable to heat in both acid and alkaline conditions. Calcium pantothenate is the stable form. Cooking, milling and food processing will readily destroy this vitamin.

□*Overdosing and toxicity* None. Some people may experience slight diarrhoea when taking large doses in excess of 2 g per day.

□*RDA* None recognized in UK. USA 4 to 7 mg. Barton Wright recommends everyone on a Western diet should take 50 mg as a supplement every day

□*Bibliography Arthritis: Cause and Control,* E.C. Barton Wright (Bunterbird Limited, London, 1975).

Pantothenic acid content of foods
in mg per 100 g

* *best sources*

wheat bran	2.4
rye flour	1.0
rye crispbread	1.1

low fat soya flour	2.1
egg custard	0.6
pancakes	0.5
dried skimmed milk	3.5
Camembert type cheese	1.4
Cheddar	0.3
Danish Blue type cheese	2.0
boiled egg	1.6
omelet	1.3
average lean back bacon/lean beef/ lamb	0.7
lean leg of pork	1.3
light chicken meat	1.2
lean roast duck	1.5
brain	1.4
roast sheep's heart	3.8
*fried lamb's kidney	5.1
stewed ox kidney	3.0
stewed pig's kidney	2.4
*fried lamb's liver	7.6
*stewed ox liver	5.7
stewed pig's liver	4.6
*fried chicken liver	5.5
steamed plaice	0.70
fried herring	0.88
fried mackerel	0.7
fresh salmon (cooked)	1.8
canned salmon	0.5
sardines	0.5
canned tuna	0.42
crab	0.60
lobster	1.63
raw oysters	0.50
fried cod's roe	2.6
boiled broad beans	3.8
boiled broccoli tops	0.7
raw cauliflower	0.60
raw mushrooms	2.0
fried mushrooms	1.4
raw tomatoes	0.33
canned tomatoes	0.20
dried raw apricots	0.70
dates	0.80
*watermelon	1.55

almonds (raw)	0.47
roasted almonds	0.25
chestnuts	0.47
dried yeast	11.0

Cooking and processing destroys this vitamin and this is illustrated in the figures for raw and cooked mushrooms, raw and canned tomatoes. In the case of peas, raw fresh peas contain 0.75 mg, cooked peas 0.32 mg and processed peas a mere 0.08 mg (per 100 g). With by far the best sources being offal, this leaves vegetarians with the poorer sources of broad beans, raw cauliflower, mushrooms, watermelon and almonds. As losses occur during cooking, using raw foods in a salad will provide a reasonable amount of pantothenic acid. Here is a suitable selection of raw foods: raw cauliflower broken into small florets, sliced raw mushrooms, a sprinkle of slivered almonds and chopped dates. Dress with oil/vinegar dressing and season with black pepper to taste. Serve on a bed of lettuce and garnish with tomato for colour. Serve with an omelet and rye crispbread. Follow with a slice of watermelon for dessert.

Non-vegetarians can obtain a high level of pantothenic acid from a dish made with lamb's liver. Wash and dry slices of lamb's liver. Coat with flour and fry in a little sunflower oil with slices of orange. Add a little orange juice to the pan and a dash of soy sauce to strengthen the gravy. Serve with steamed broccoli tops and potatoes or boiled broad beans and rice. Follow with watermelon.

■Vitamin B6/Pyridoxine hydrochloride, pyridoxal & pyridoxamine, pyridoxal-phosphate

□*Water-soluble.*

□*Natural sources* Yeast, liver, cereals, meat, green vegetables, nuts, fresh and dried fruits.

□*Commercial forms for supplements* Pyridoxine hydrochloride is the normal form of vitamin B6 found commercially. It is usually produced synthetically, but bio-synthetic processes are sometimes used.

□*Main functions* Used to form the enzyme codecarboxylase (pyridoxal 5 phosphate) which plays a part in many major metabolic processes, including protein metabolism. It is now widely recommended for premenstrual tension and also for morning sickness in pregnancy, but this is controversial and not backed by sufficient clinical evidence. Women on the contraceptive pill often find that they require extra B6.

□*Main deficiency symptoms* Convulsions in babies, certain forms of anaemia, depression, dizziness. Nervous disorders have been associated with B6 deficiency. Skin and mouth eruptions and neuritis in the outlying body area (peripheral).

□*Co-factors* Vitamin B1, B2, pantothenic acid, linoleic acid (an essential fatty acid – vitamin F factor).

□*Stability* It is destroyed in the presence of iron, oxidizing agents and alkaline conditions. As a water soluble vitamin it will be lost in cooking water if discarded.

□*Overdosing and toxicity* In high doses, 500 mg daily, some nervous problems have been reported. All problems are reversed as soon as the vitamin is stopped. It is not recommended to be taken in high doses for prolonged periods except under professional supervision.

□*RDA* 2 to 2.2 mg. Up to 100 mg daily is often used by women on the contraceptive pill and this would appear to be a safe long-term regime.

□*Bibliography* *The Vitamins*, vol. 2, W. H. Sebrell & R.S. Harris (Academia, New York, 1968), pp. 1-117.

■Vitamins B10 and B11

Two factors reported to be necessary for growth and feathering of chicks. (See Merck Index, Tenth Edition, 9821.)
No structures proposed and so no official vitamin status applies.

■Vitamin B12/cyanocobalamin, the cobalamins, hydroxocobalamin

□*Water-soluble* (slightly).

□*Natural sources* Produced by bacteria in the intestines but cannot be absorbed at that point. Liver, meat, eggs, fish. Vegetarians and vegans may become deficient and a precaution for those following these meat-excluding diets would be a supplement of B12 to yield about 10 to 50 mcg daily. Alfalfa, comfrey and spirulina are weak vegetable sources of vitamin B12.

□*Commercial forms*   Cyanocobalamin is the usual form of B12 and is produced by fermentation processes. Hydroxocobalamin is the form used widely in injections to treat patients with pernicious anaemia.

□*Main functions*   Important in iron metabolism, nerve condition and cell life.

□*Main deficiency symptoms*   Pernicious anaemia, fatigue, depression, nervousness and loss of reflex responses.

□*Co-vitamins*   B complex, especially folic acid.

□*Stability*   Very stable in supplements. In cooking, about 30% of the vitamin may be lost.

□*Overdosing and toxicity*   B12 is not toxic, but if supplements are used it is important to tell your doctor if you are to have a blood test. B12 interferes with some tests and could lead to a misdiagnosis. Your doctor will tell you to stop all supplements before having the test. B12 is administered by injection for pernicious anaemia – the classic deficiency disease of B12. This is caused by lack of an enzyme in the stomach called intrinsic factor which is essential for aborption of B12 from food; thus supplements by mouth would be ineffective. B12 from supplements is absorbed by normal people and it is quite a common mistake to read that B12 is not absorbed by mouth because of the existence of injections. Writers forget that the anaemia is caused by lack of intrinsic factor not B12 in the diet. Some nutritionists believe that pure B12 supplements should be sucked rather than swallowed because substantial absorption can take place through the mouth mucosa.

□*RDA*   3 mcg. Supplements 5 to 50 mcg.

Vitamin B12 content of foods
in mcg per 100 g

* *best sources*

grains, cereals, bread, fruit and vegetables	0
fresh milk	0.3
dried skimmed milk	3.0
butter	*trace*
Camembert type cheese	1.2
Cheddar	1.5
cottage cheese	0.5
yoghurt	*trace*

egg	1.7
raw egg yolk	4.9
bacon	*trace*
lean beef	2.0
lean lamb	2.0
lean pork	3.0
chicken	*trace*
lean duck	3.0
dark turkey meat	3.0
stewed rabbit	12.0
brain	9.0
heart	13 – 15
*fried lamb's kidney	79.0
*stewed ox kidney	31.0
stewed pig's kidney	15.0
*fried calf liver	87.0
*fried chicken liver	49.0
*stewed ox liver	110.0
stewed pig's liver	26.0
corned beef	2.0
ham	*trace*
baked cod	2.0
steamed haddock	1.0
fried herring	11.0
fried mackerel	9.0
fresh salmon	6.0
*sardines	28.0
tuna in oil	5.0
crab, lobster	*trace*
raw oysters	15.0
fried cod's roe	11.0

■Vitamin B13

Orotic Acid. Whey factor. Normally found in food supplements combined with minerals, for example calcium orotate, iron orotate, zinc orotate.

Not an officially recognized vitamin, therefore there is no RDA.

□*Natural sources*   Milk.

□*Synthetic forms*   Several methods of synthesis are known using natural starting materials such as urea. The amounts present in milk are too small to be extracted commercially.

Main functions Mineral transport in the body. A natural chelator (mineral binder). Orotates may help gout sufferers.

□*Deficiencies* Not known.

□*Co-factors* Essential minerals.

□*Overdosing and toxicity* None reported.

□*Stability* Very stable.

□*Research and Bibliography* Moruzzi et al., *Biochem. Z, 333,* 318 (1960); Manna, Hauge. *J. Biol. Chem., 202,* 91 (1953).

■ Vitamin B15/Pangamic acid

Mixture of calcium gluconate and N N dimethylglycine or di-isopropylamine dichloroacetate. Not an officially recognized vitamin.

□*Water-soluble*

□*Natural sources* The only thing that is certain about this substance is its presence somewhere in apricot kernels because that is where its discoverer E.T. Krebs (*Int. Rec. Med.,* 164, 18, 1951) found it.

□*Commercial forms* Synthetic mixtures of above.

□*Main functions* None recognized, but enthusiasts have claimed enhanced athletic performance and aid for heart and circulatory diseases. The Russians are said to have given combinations of B15 and herbs to their successful athletes and astronauts. Muhammed Ali, the heavyweight boxing champion, claimed to have used it to help him win a famous boxing match against George Foreman, held in Zaire. Proponents say it is a methyl donor like choline.

□*Deficiency symptoms* None recognized.

□*Co-factors* Vitamins E, C, B-complex, particularly choline, another methyl donor.

□*Stability* Since its structure is in doubt, no details are available but the commercial forms as marketed are stable.

□*Overdosing and toxicity* The controversy surrounding B15 has led its denigrators to find toxic effects. These are really little better founded than the beneficial claims. No really independent research has been carried out. In the USA the main manufacturers of the original B15 now sell a product just containing N N dimethylglycine but make no claims. The packaging of the product and its appearance is very similar to the original B15 product. We keep an open mind, but would not really accept either side of the substance's story. Certainly calcium gluconate is totally safe, and this appears to form over 50% of B15.

□*RDA*   None. Supplements containing 50 mg have been sold in the USA to millions of people for over 15 years.

■Vitamin B17/Amygdalin, Laetrile, Nitrolisides

Not an officially recognized vitamin.

□*Water-soluble*

□*Natural sources*   Apricots and peach kernels, bitter almonds.

□*Commercial forms*   Pure Amygdalin extracted from apricot kernels.

□*Main functions*   Probably the most controversial nutritional substance of the last forty years. Krebs attributed the freedom from cancer in the Hunza tribe in the Himalayas to their diet high in apricots. He proposed the active anti-cancer principle to be laetrile, later identified as amygdalin. No subsequent scientific evidence has been provided to back Krebs' claim, yet vast numbers of cancer sufferers in the USA have tried this substance, and a great many books about the laetrile treatment exist. We would not claim amygdalin as a cancer cure, but used within a proper holistic treatment regime it may have a positive role to play for some patients.

□*Deficiency symptoms*   None recognized.

□*Co-vitamins*   Vitamin A, selenium, vitamin E and vitamin C – preferably neutralized or buffered.

□*Stability*   Very stable.

□*Overdosing and toxicity*   Amygdalin contains the cyanide grouping within its structure. This cyanide is not free and requires the action of an enzyme to release it. The proponents of its use in cancer state that the cyanide is only liberated in tumour cells where it kills the malignancy. The opponents say this is nonsense and science is on their side. The problem with laetrile is that the cyanide can be liberated in the stomach and cause death. The opponents of laetrile treatment say that it is worthless as a cancer treatment. Perhaps the following facts are worth recording so that readers can make up their own minds.

Lethal dose of free cyanide is 250 mg (Martindale, Extra Pharmacopoeia, 28th Edition, 1983).

Content of bound cyanide in a 250 mg tablet of amygdalin (the strongest product normally available) 13 mg. Dose of 20 tablets at one time would be lethal if 100% of the cyanide were released – a most unlikely situation. 20 tablets would never be taken at a single time as most of the laetrile therapists recommend a maximum dose at any one time of 500 mg – never exceeding 2 g per day.

Content of bound cyanide in 25 mg amygdalin tablet is 1.3 mg and some 200 tablets would need to be taken at a single time to approach the lethal dose of cyanide if it were all released. Certain common over-the-counter drugs such as aspirins and para-cetamols would be more toxic than this.

Patients have died in the USA using amygdalin in high doses, but equally many more have died using some of the powerful drugs used as anti-tumour agents. In the UK all amygdalin preparations are available on doctor's prescription.

□*RDA*   None.

■Vitamin Bc/Folic acid or vitamin M

Also known by complex chemical names, one of the shortest of which is pteroylglutamic acid.

□*Water-soluble*   slightly.

□*Natural sources*   Eggs, liver, leafy green vegetables, milk, grains.

□*Commercial forms for supplements*   Folic acid may be synthesized chemically. In natural sources it is combined with protein structures closely allied with glutamic acid.

□*Main functions*   Important in many enzyme systems, including the construction of proteins and DNA. In preventing anaemia a balance between folic acid and vitamin B12 must be maintained.

□*Main deficiency symptoms*   Megaloblastic anaemia, digestive problems, growth retardation, tongue inflammation, memory impairment and greying of hair.

□*Co-factors*   B-complex, especially B12, vitamin C.

□*Stability*   Cooking may deprive food of up to 90% of its folic acid content. Boiling green vegetables will leach out the folic acid, so do not throw away the water. Heavy metals, such as iron, copper and manganese, will aid its destruction. Several drugs destroy it in the body including the anti-malarial pyrimethamine and some anti-convulsants such as phenytoin.

□*Overdosing and toxicity*   Folic acid is taken in relatively small doses. 15 mg daily is considered a large dose, but even at that level it is non-toxic. The real problem with it relates to its effect on vitamin B12. People with pernicious anaemia (B12 deficiency) should not take folic acid because it lowers the B12 blood levels even more. If you are taking supplements and have blood tests you must inform your doctor of this. If you take concentrated folic acid supplements be sure to take adequate B12 too. In B-complexes an appropriate balance of these items is usually built into the formulas, but this is not a 1:1 ratio.

□*RDA*   400 mcg.

NOTE: A close relative of folic acid is folinic acid (see page XXX).

Folic acid content of foods
in mcg per 100 g

These figures apply to the total amount of folic acid in the foods. Some of this is termed 'free' and some 'bound'. The free is more readily lost in cooking but both types are available to the body for nutritional purposes.

* *best sources*

wheat germ	330
wheat bran	260
wholewheat flour	57
wholewheat bread	39
plain white flour	19
white bread	27
raw oatmeal	60
rye flour	78
* All-Bran	100
rye crispbread	40
dried skimmed milk	21
Camembert type cheese	60

Danish Blue type cheese	50
Cheddar	20
cottage cheese	9
yoghurt	2
raw egg	25
omelet	22
lean meat	
topside (beef)	17
leg of lamb	4
leg of pork	7
fried lamb's kidney	79
* fried calf liver	320
* fried chicken liver	500
* fried lamb's liver	240
* stewed ox liver	290
stewed pig's liver	110
baked cod	12
crab	20
boiled beetroot	50
raw beetroot	90
* boiled broccoli tops	110
* raw Brussels sprouts	110
cooked Brussels sprouts	87
raw red cabbage	90
boiled spring cabbage	50
boiled winter cabbage	35
old raw carrots	15
raw cauliflower	39
cucumber	16
* raw endive	330
lettuce	34
raw mushrooms	23
cooked onions	8
* boiled fresh or frozen peas	78
processed peas	3
raw or cooked green pepper	11
old, raw, baked potatoes	10
new boiled potatoes	10
radishes	24
* boiled spinach	140
boiled swede	21
raw tomatoes	28
canned tomatoes	25
* boiled turnip tops	110
avocado pears	66

raw bananas	22
dates	21
melon	30
orange	37
strawberries	20
* almonds	96
hazel nuts	72
* fresh peanuts	110
walnuts	66
tomato purée	140
yeast extract spread	1010
meat extract spread	1040
dried yeast	4000

Although the last three items on this list are very high in folic acid they are only eaten in very small quantities. The easiest way to ensure a good, constant supply of this vitamin is to make sure your diet includes a good helping of cooked green vegetables every day. Spinach and broccoli tops are particularly good value.

■Vitamin Bt/L-Carnitine

□*Water-soluble* .

□*Natural sources*   Striated muscle, meat. It is produced in the body's own metabolic processes and is not an officially recognized vitamin.

□*Commercial forms supplements*   May be synthesized from several starting chemicals including epichlorohydrin and aminohydroxy butyric acid.

□*Main functions*   Involved in the metabolism of essential fatty acids. Burns fats. Stimulates secretion of gastric and pancreatic enzymes, so speeding digestive processes. Aid to heart and circulatory problems. Lowers cholesterol and increases HDL (High Density Lipo-protein).

□*Deficiency symptoms*   None reported. Some nutrition magazines have reported that muscle weakness and degeneration has been reversed or improved by using supplements of L-Carnitine. Slow brain function has also been helped, according to these sources.

□*Co-vitamins*   Essential fatty acids, vitamin E and vitamin C.

□*Stability*   Very stable.

□*Overdosing and toxicity*   D-Carnitine is not as well tolerated as a supplement as L-carnitine. Diarrhoea occurs at high dose levels – in excess of 4 g daily.

□*RDA*   None officially. In supplements 250 to 1000 mg daily.

■Para aminobenzoic acid (vitamin Bx)

Not an accepted vitamin, frequently called PABA, and even H3 factor.

□*Water-soluble*   .

□*Natural sources*   Yeast, liver, wheat germ, brans, milk.

□*Commercial forms used in supplements*   All commercial PABA is prepared synthetically by fairly simple chemical methods.

□*Main functions*   No convincing scientific proof is available, although it is recommended variously for preventing grey hair colour, keeping young and in good general health. A form of PABA is used in sunscreen creams and is useful for this purpose. It is usually included in comprehensive B-complex supplements as a co-factor.

□*Main deficiency symptoms*   None officially recognized. It is probably useful as a co-factor in helping the B-vitamins work more efficiently and may therefore be associated with general B vitamin deficiency states.

□*Co-factors*   B complex.

□*Stability*   Very stable, except in the presence of ferric iron and other oxidizing agents.

□*RDA*   None officially. In B complex supplements 10 to 100 mg is usually found.

If you are taking a course of sulpha drugs for an infection, PABA should not be taken as its presence will interfere with the action of those drugs. Sulpha drugs act by mimicking PABA in the body. Bacteria depend upon PABA for their survival, and when they absorb the Sulpha drug instead they die. This is the reason that many authorities limit the amount of PABA allowed in food supplements. We advise everyone taking supplements to inform their doctors if they are using vitamins generally when seeking advice on illnesses.

It must be remembered that as Sulpha drugs kill unfriendly invading bacteria, so they destroy the friendly microflora of the intestine. During the recovery phase of an illness where Sulpha drugs have been used, it is always a good idea to ensure that you use a supplement which contains PABA so that the friendly microflora can re-establish themselves quickly.

H3's youth factor provides an interesting sidelight on PABA. Professor Aslan in Bucharest in the 1950s proposed that procaine had youth-giving properties. This substance breaks down in the body to two substances, one of which is PABA. Procaine is a prescription controlled drug in Britain, so in order to take advantage of the magic term H3 many manufacturers just add PABA to their products. Aslan's work has remained unconfirmed to this day, but injections containing procaine as well as tablets and capsules providing the H3 factor still have many devotees among those searching for eternal youth.

■Choline

Occurs naturally in lecithin. It is not a vitamin but is associated with the B-complex as it occurs in foodstuffs rich in B vitamins.

□*Water-soluble* A very hygroscopic material – readily absorbs water from the air.

□*Natural sources* Lecithin, brewer's yeast, soya beans, egg yolk, legumes.

□*Commercial forms for supplements* Choline used in supplements is derived synthetically from trimethylamine and ethylene oxide. The chloride or tartrate is the usual source used. The tartrate contains approximately 50% choline, whilst the chloride is much richer – at over 80% – but much more hygroscopic and therefore less suitable for preparing tablets and capsules.

□*Main functions* As a methyldonor in metabolism and forms part of the neuro-transmitter substance acetylcholine. Found throughout nerve tissue. It has been described as a lipotropic substance, that is fat resistant – thus helping to stop fatty degeneration of organs like blood vessels and liver.

□*Main deficiency symptoms* Intolerance to fats, poor nerve transmission with associated general health problems. Deficiency is unlikely except in severe starvation situations. Choline can be made by the body using the amino acid Methionine derived from digestion of proteins.

□*Co-factors* B-complex, especially inositol and the polyunsaturates (essential fatty acids).

□*Stability*   Stable, but in supplements choline compounds cause problems because they readily absorb moisture from the air and may cause tablets to become damp. This dampness may lead other vitamins in the supplement to deteriorate, but the choline would retain its integrity as a compound.

□*Overdosing and toxicity*   More than 5 g daily may cause gastric discomfort, diarrhoea and nausea.

□*RDA*   None officially given as it is not considered an essential nutrient. In supplements, 50 to 1000 mg are taken. Beware of products labelled with a content of choline where it is the bitartrate which is the stated strength – only half labelled strength is really choline in such cases. Look for the words 'Choline bitartrate' or 'Choline' on products.

■Folinic acid

A relative of folic acid, to which it is converted with the aid of vitamin C in the body. It is used as an antidote for folic acid deficiency caused by certain drugs which are folate antagonists (enemies).

□*Natural sources*   Brewer's yeast.

□*Synthetic forms*   Calcium folinate. It is not found in food supplements. It is solely used in fairly high doses of 15 mg as an antidote to the anti-folate drugs. Since it is so closely related to folic acid, to which it is converted by the body, it will have the same general functions and deficiency symptoms (see page 85).

■Inositol

Occurs naturally in lecithin. It is not a vitamin, but like choline, it is found in association with B-complex vitamins in foodstuffs so is usually considered as a nutrient within that family.

□*Water-soluble*

□*Natural sources*   Lecithin, brewer's yeast, whole grains (especially brans), meat, nuts and fruits.

□*Commercial forms for supplements*   Commercially obtained from maize by extraction processes.

□*Main functions*   Controversial ideas put forward include prevention of baldness, prevention of overweight and heart disease. None of these ideas has any valid scientific proof.

Vitamins

□*Deficiency symptoms*   Poor health in general, but no specific symptom yet discovered.

□*Co-factors*   B-complex, especially choline and polyunsaturates. (Vitamin F factors.)

□*Stability*   Very stable.

□*Overdosing and toxicity*   None. Indeed inositol has been proposed as a good chewable base for vitamin tablets. It has a very sweet taste. It is expensive, currently some 50 times more costly than sugar and only marginally sweeter, so one would find it difficult to discover any commercial supplements using it as a chewable base.

□*RDA*   None. We suggest a balance with choline itself, not Choline bitartrate (see page 90).

■Vitamin C

Ascorbic acid, L-ascorbic acid, cevitamic acid, also available as various mineral ascorbates, e.g. calcium ascorbate.

□*Water-soluble*   .

□*Natural sources*   Fresh fruit and vegetables, especially citrus fruits and green peppers. Rosehips. Acerola cherry berries grown in Puerto Rico are one of the richest natural sources. Potatoes.

□*Synthetic forms*   The ascorbic acid of commerce is all synthesized using a basic fermentation process starting with a natural starch, e.g. corn or potato. Powders labelled 'natural' are invariably boosted with processed vitamin C to ensure that they meet label potencies.

□*Main functions*   Anti-scurvy – the classic vitamin deficiency disease of sailors in the middle ages (see Introduction, page 4). Disease resistance, building collagen and intercellular material. Healing of wounds. It also acts as an antioxidant and is often formulated with other antioxidant nutrients such as vitamin E, selenium and glutathione.

□*Main deficiency symptoms*   Bleeding gums, poor resistance to colds, anaemia (its connection with folinic acid to folate conversion, and also its need in iron metabolism), connective tissue breakdown, blood vessel weakness, broken capillaries on skin surface.

□*Co-factors*   Whilst most vitamins and minerals work with vitamin C, those especially connected include vitamin A, B-complex for stress, and bioflavonoids – the so called vitamin P factors.

□*Stability*   Up to 50% is lost in cooking – excessive stirring and boiling makes matters even worse. Oxidizing agents such as nitrates and ferric iron salts break it down rapidly. Smoking is said to destroy 25 mg per cigarette smoked. Tablets darken on storage and packages should be kept tightly closed and away from direct light to preserve product potency. Some drugs seem to destroy the vitamin, and these include aspirin and cortisone.

□*Overdosing and toxicity*   Too much can lead to hyperacidity with stomach discomfort. It is better to use buffered or neutralized products, such as those made with calcium ascorbate or combined with a neutralizing agent such as dolomite, especially if high doses (over 1 g daily) are to be taken for a long period. The calcium or magnesium ascorbates are preferred to the sodium form (see mineral sodium, page 130). Large doses may cause diarrhoea and kidney stones of calcium oxalate. Over 600 mg daily is slightly diuretic. We would not advise more than 3 g per day except under professional supervision. People can develop tolerance to large doses and develop a deficiency if the amount of daily supplementation is suddenly reduced.

□*RDA*   50 to 60 mg daily. 10 mg daily is said to be enough to prevent clinical scurvy. Pregnancy and lactation put greater demands on requirements and probably a useful supplementary insurance would be 250 mg daily for everyone.

Vitamin C content of foods
in mg per 100 g

* *best sources*

fresh cow's milk	1.5
dried skimmed milk	6.0
human milk	3.7
single cream	1.2
yoghurt	0.4
brain	17
fried lamb's kidney	9
fried calf liver	13
fried chicken liver	13
fried lamb's liver	12
stewed ox liver	15
stewed pig's liver	9
fried lamb's sweetbreads	18
fried cod's roe	26

asparagus	20
runner beans	20
broad beans	15
* cooked broccoli tops	34
* raw Brussels sprouts	90
cooked Brussels sprouts	40
* raw red cabbage	55
spring cabbage (cooked)	25
raw white cabbage	40
old raw carrots	6
cooked old carrots	4
* raw cauliflower	60
cooked cauliflower	20
raw celery	7
raw cucumber	8
endive	12
boiled leeks	15
raw mushrooms	3
mustard and cress	40
* raw spring onions	25
cooked onion	6
cooked parsnips	10
boiled fresh peas	15
canned processed peas	*trace*
split peas	*trace*
* raw green pepper	100
cooked old potatoes	16
new boiled potatoes	18
* raw radishes	25
* boiled spinach	25
* boiled spring greens	30
boiled swede	17
raw tomatoes	20
boiled turnips	17
* raw watercress	60
eating apple	3
baked apple	14
fresh raw apricots	7
dried apricots	*trace*
avocado pears	15
raw bananas	10
stewed blackberries	14
fresh cherries	5
* stewed blackcurrants	140

stewed gooseberries	28
grapes	4
* raw grapefruit	40
canned grapefruit juice	28
canned grapefruit	30
* canned guavas	180
fresh lemon juice	50
raw lychees	40
raw mango	30
melon	25
watermelon	5
* fresh oranges	50
canned orange juice	35
passion fruit	20
peaches	8
pears	3
* fresh pineapple	25
canned pineapple juice	8
plums	3
* raspberries	25
* strawberries	60
tangerines	30
canned tomato juice	20
tomato purée	100

Although we tend to think of vitamin C as being only in fruit, it is also in vegetables, offal and milk. Cooking and processing tend to destroy this vitamin and you can see this illustrated in the list, e.g. the 15 mg in fresh boiled peas reduces to only a trace in processed peas. Fruit juices contain less than the fresh fruit. Cauliflower loses ⅔ of its vitamin C after cooking.

Dried fruit contains only a trace or no vitamin C at all. Nuts have only a trace and wines and spirits contain none at all in spite of many of them being made from fruit. The poorest sources are cereals, grains, bread, cheese, meat [except for some offal], fish, eggs, fats and oils.

Here is a salad which is very high in vitamin C. If prepared just before eating, the value of this important vitamin will be at its maximum.

High vitamin C winter salad   for 1 person

Mix the following together in a salad bowl   3 raw Brussels sprouts [shredded] or 1 red cabbage leaf [shredded], 3 or 4 cauliflower florets [chopped], ¼ pkt mustard and cress, ¼ of a green pepper [chopped], 1 raw spring onion [chopped], 3 or 4 radishes [sliced] and 1 tomato [chopped]. Sprinkle with ½ teaspoon sugar and 2 grinds of black pepper. Mix 3 teaspoons sunflower oil with 1 teaspoon fresh lemon juice [in a cup] and pour over the salad. Turn over with two spoons to mix thoroughly and serve.

For a very high vitamin C meal serve the salad with homemade chicken liver pâté [see p.69], on wholewheat toast. Follow with a dessert of stewed blackcurrants or fresh orange segments mixed with a passion fruit or fresh strawberries.

■ Vitamin D

There are several forms known either by chemical names or more simply as D1, D2, D3 and D4. The only two which concern us are D2 and D3. All have the same biological action in preventing the bone-softening disease Rickets. D2 is usually known as calciferol or ergocalciferol, whilst D3 is cholecalciferol, and this is the accepted standard vitamin D substance.

□*Oil-soluble*

□*Natural sources*   Fish oils, egg yolks, organ meat, bone meal, milk. Naturally occurring steroids in the body are converted by sunlight to active vitamin D, so sunlight is a source.

□*Commercial forms for supplements*   D2 ergocalciferol is a synthetic form produced by irradiation of ergosterol (no connection with the ergot alkaloids used in drugs for migraine and assisting childbirth). D3 is the natural form of vitamin D, but all commercial D3 is produced synthetically by irradiation of 7-dehydrocholesterol – its natural provitamin.

□*Main functions*   Building healthy bones with the aid of the minerals calcium and phosphorus.

□*Main deficiency symptoms*   Softening of bones, rickets, softening of teeth, nervousness, insomnia, diarrhoea, burning sensation in mouth and throat said to be sub-clinical indications of deficiency.

□*Co-vitamins*   Vitamin A, calcium and phosphorus. This vitamin always figures in health vitamin supplements, even the simplest ones such as Vitaminorum BPC.

□*Stability*   Vitamin D content of foodstuffs is stable to cooking. Pure synthetic vitamin Ds are not stable in moist air. Specially pre-pared powders which are very stable are available for preparing supplements and fortifying foods but preparations must be kept com-pletely dry.

□*Overdosing and toxicity* Vitamin D has been termed a hormone rather than a vitamin by some scientists because of its very potent biological activity. It is toxic in regular doses of 25,000 iu daily, and the maximum daily supplementation should not exceed 2000 iu except under professional supervision. Symptoms of overdosing include anorexia, nausea, sickness, weight loss, diarrhoea, sweating, extreme thirst and vertigo.

□*RDA* 200 to 400 iu. More is seldom required in supplements. The International Unit is based upon the element of activity of cholecalciferol vitamin D3, one unit being equivalent to 0.025 mcg of D3. All preparations of vitamin D must be labelled with reference to that standard.

Vitamin D content of foods
in mcg per 100 g

* *best sources*

shortbread	0.23
rich fruit cake	1.14
sponge cake with fat	1.59
shortcrust pastry	1.38
butter	0.76
egg	1.76
raw egg yolk	5.0
* cod liver oil	210.0
margarine	7.94
vegetable oils	0
meat	*trace*
calf liver	0.25
lamb's liver	0.50
stewed ox liver	1.13
pig's liver	1.13
* grilled herring	25.0
* fried mackerel	15.4
* pilchards	8.0
fresh salmon	*trace*
* canned salmon	12.5
* sardines	7.5
tuna in oil	5.8
crustacea and molluscs	*trace*
fried cod's roe	2.0
fruit and vegetables	0

Vitamin D is added to margarine during processing. Cod liver oil is widely used to supplement the diet with this vitamin which is not found in a great number of foods.

□*High vitamin D recipe*

Baked herrings

A very inexpensive and simple main course, high in vitamin D. For each person allow 1 medium sized potato, 1 filleted and cleaned herring (fresh), 1 good pinch each of marjoram and thyme (dried), black pepper, good squeeze fresh lemon juice, ½ medium sized onion cut into rings and a little butter.

Preheat the oven at Gas Mark 5 (190°C/375°F). Grease a baking dish. Peel the potato, part boil for 5 minutes and strain. Cut into thin slices and use half to line the dish. Lay the herring fillets on top and sprinkle with the herbs and lemon juice. Cover with the onion slices and the remaining potato slices. Dot with small pieces of butter and season to taste with black pepper. Bake in the oven for about 35 to 40 minutes and serve immediately with plenty of wholewheat bread (dry), and green salad.

■Vitamin E/D-alpha tocopherol

Other tocopherols, including beta and gamma, are sometimes included in whole natural vitamin E products. The esters, based on acetic acid (tocopheryl acetate) and succinic acid (tocopheryl succinate), are used in supplements because of their stability.

□*Oil-soluble*

□*Natural sources*　Soya beans, wheat germ, sprouting seeds, dark green vegetables, eggs, nuts, vegetable oils.

□*Synthetic forms*　Most commercial natural vitamin E is prepared by extraction processes from soya bean oil. The pure oil is converted to suitable Esters by the appropriate organic acids, e.g. acetic acid for tocopheryl acetate. There is a dl alpha tocopherol as well and the letters dl indicate a mixture of the natural d form and the synthetic l form. Products containing dl vitamin E are considered wholly synthetic and are much cheaper than those produced from the natural extracted d alpha form.

□*Main functions*　Antioxidant with protective properties on cells. Its role in curing impotence and female infertility is unproven. Benefits to heart and circulatory problems, as well as injury healing, whilst controversial are more firmly based. Much research is currently being carried out on this vitamin in connection with varicose veins, phlebitis, menstrual and menopausal problems. In creams, vitamin E may help heal stretch marks and scars, but long term regular application is essential. Internal use is also recommended to complement external preparations.

☐*Main deficiency symptoms* None really accepted by science. Many nutritionists believe sexual problems, including impotency in men and infertility and miscarriages in women, are in part caused by vitamin E deficiency. Heart disease and muscle wasting are also mentioned, as is poor skin and hair condition. Lack of antioxidants like vitamin E will certainly shorten cell life. If people take diets high in polyunsaturates extra vitamin E is required.

☐*Co-factors* Selenium, vitamin C, polyunsaturated fatty acids.

☐*Stability* Very stable in the ester form, but the tocopherols themselves are destroyed in the presence of air. Hence only acetates or succinates are found in commercial supplements. Some nutritionists recommend iron supplements should be taken apart from vitamin E, but the evidence for this is based on research involving premature babies and has not been duplicated in children, babies or adults.

☐*Overdosing and toxicity* If high doses are taken without gradual build-up over a 14 day period blood pressure may increase. Very high doses may cause gastric discomfort and fatigue.

☐*RDA* Not officially recognized in the United Kingdom. Elsewhere 10 iu. The international unit (iu) of activity is equivalent to that of 1 mg of synthetic dl alpha tocopherol acetate. Natural d alpha forms are more potent, but controversy surrounds this claim. At present the figure for units of activity for natural d alpha tocopherol acetate is 1.36 times that for synthetic dl form per mg.

Vitamin E content of foods

in mg per 100 g

* *best sources*	
* wheat germ	11.0
raw oatmeal	0.8
rye flour	0.8
All-Bran	2.0
Puffed Wheat	1.7
muesli	3.2
Weetabix	1.8

rich, iced fruit cake	2.4
sponge cake with fat	2.7
shortcrust pastry	1.4
butter	2.0
eggs	1.6
raw egg yolk	4.6
cod liver oil	20.0
* margarine	8.0
tuna in oil	6.3
lobster	1.5
mussels	1.2
fried cod's roe	6.9
asparagus	1.3
broccoli tops (boiled)	1.1
raw Brussels sprouts	1.0
raw parsley	1.8
boiled spinach	2.0
raw tomatoes	1.2
avocado pear	3.2
raw blackberries	3.5
* almonds	20.0
brazils	6.5
* hazel nuts	21.0
peanuts	8.1
walnuts	0.8
tomato purée	6.9

In vegetable oils the vitamin E varies considerably from one oil to the next. The vitamin E is classed as active tocopheryls and there are three main types – alpha, gamma and delta. Of these three the most active is alpha tocopheryl. The following three small charts help to illustrate the carrying amounts of vitamin E found in oils.

Oils	active alpha tocopheryl (vitamin E)
maize	11.2
olive	5.1
palm	25.6
peanut	13.0
rapeseed	18.4

Oils (contd)	active gamma tocopheryl (vitamin E)
safflowerseed	38.7
soybean	10.1
sunflowerseed	48.7
wheat germ	133.0

Oils	active gamma tocopheryl (vitamin E)
cottonseed	38.7
maize	60.2
palm	31.6
rapeseed	38.0
safflowerseed	17.4
soybean	59.3

Oils	delta tocopheryl (vitamin E)
maize	1.8
palm	7.0
safflowerseed	24.0
soybean	26.4
wheat germ	27.1

Muesli containing hazel nuts and almonds as well as wheat germ would seem to be a good source of vitamin E that can be taken regularly. The use of margarine daily will also help with a regular intake of this vitamin. Although the vitamin E content of the vegetables in the list seems quite low, they can be eaten in fairly large quantities which makes them a good source, in spite of low fat content. Best vegetable oil to use for cooking and salads in relation to vitamin is sunflowerseed oil. Choose ones which are very pale in colour as the darker yellow ones are showing signs of being stale. Best oils to buy are in tins as they are not then prone to deterioration caused by sunlight.

■Vitamin F

A term not scientifically accepted but which many nutritionists persist in using when referring to a group of essential fatty acids known as the polyunsaturates. These include (omega 6 series) linoleic acid, gamma linolenic acid (GLA); (omega 3 series) eicosapentaenoic acid (EPA) and docosahexanoic acid (DHA).

□*Oil-soluble.*

□*Natural sources*   Omega 6 series: sunflower oil, safflower oil, wheat germ oil, corn oil and evening primrose oil. Omega 3 series: fish oils.

□*Commercial forms*   All are natural oils and the richest sources are used in supplements, e.g. evening primrose oil for omega 6 and fish oils for omega 3. Synthetic methods of production are known but are more expensive than natural oils of similar potency.

□*Main functions*   The formation of active biological substances in the body called prostaglandins which control blood clotting. Polyunsaturates are also claimed to lower blood cholesterol levels and protect against heart attacks and high blood pressure.

There have been many claims about the benefits of polyunsaturates. The western diet is too rich in saturated fats and our bodies need to obtain more polyunsaturated fat because this forms the muscle structures and cell walls. If no polyunsaturates are available the body uses saturated fatty acid for this purpose and structural weaknesses ensue. Both sorts of fat are needed in our bodies, and a balance between the two of them is important. Research into the EPA series (omega 3) has shown definite benefits as regards lowering cholesterol levels in the blood using supplements.

Research using omega 6 series evening primrose oil has shown a very wide spectrum of benefits but few scientists accept this research. Successful use of evening primrose for premenstrual tension, rheumatoid arthritis, multiple sclerosis, eczema, food allergy, and hyperactivity in children has been reported, but double blind studies using sunflower oil or safflower oil as placebo have not been reported in these conditions. One trial used mineral oil as placebo – a substance which exacerbates the nutritional status of people by removing the oily vitamins A, D, E and K from the body. We are not surprised that people on the evening primrose oil did better. Evening primrose oil is considered superior to sunflower oil because it contains GLA. This substance is a step nearer the prostaglandin substance needed by the body than the linolenic acid of sunflower oil. The theory is that many people cannot convert Linolenic acid to prostaglandins because their bodies cannot convert linolenic acid to GLA. Therefore, giving these people GLA will bring them back to health. The trouble is that there is no evidence at all that the body can use GLA directly, and the reaction linolenic acid – GLA – prostaglandin is a theory, not a fact. The GLA step may not take place at all. So if you are one of those using expensive evening primrose oil, try sunflower oil or safflower oil – you might find them just as good.

□*Main deficiency symptoms*   High cholesterol level in the blood, dry skin, brittle hair, eczema.

□*Co-factors*   Vitamin E.

□*Stability*   Polyunsaturated fatty acids deteriorate when exposed to the air and become rancid. In supplements, vitamin E is added to protect them. It is best to store the pure oils in a cool dark place and keep the bottle or container tightly closed. If you are cooking with polyunsaturated oils it is best to use once only since heating will cause the oil to deteriorate.

□*Overdosing and toxicity*   None. Several ounces of sunflower oil could be used daily, but keep a balance of your fats saturated to polyunsaturated. A maximum of 10% of total daily calories should be from polyunsaturates.

□*RDA*   None. It is recommended that there should be a balance between dietary intake of polyunsaturated fatty acids and saturated fatty acids. More than 1% of total calorie intake should be polyunsaturated fatty acids (vitamin F).

□*Bibliography*   *Essential Fatty Acids and Prostaglandins*, R. J. Holman (Pergamon Press, New York, 1982).

■Vitamin H/Biotin, Biocytin

□*Water-soluble* (very slightly).

□*Natural sources*   Brewer's yeast, egg yolks, whole grains, organ meats, especially liver and kidney. Also produced in the body by healthy intestinal flora.

□*Commercial forms for supplements*   Biotin is prepared synthetically, but pure material can be obtained from natural origins. Biotin in natural form can be isolated from yeast.

□*Main functions*   It acts as a vital coenzyme for protein and carbohydrate metabolic processes. It is found in every cell and is termed a growth factor.

□*Main deficiency symptoms*   Retardation of growth, depression, general fatigue and skin eruptions.

□*Co-vitamins*   B complex, folic acid, vitamin B12 and vitamin C.

□*Stability*   Generally very stable. Biotin is inactivated by avidin, a substance occurring in raw egg whites. Diets rich in raw egg whites may lead to a deficiency.

□*Overdosing and toxicity*　Biotin is a very expensive substance and pure supplements exceeding a strength of 1 mg per dose are rare. No toxic level is known.

□*RDA*　100 to 300 mcg.

□*Bibliography*　*Vitamins and Coenzymes*, A. F. Wagner and K. Folkes (Wiley, New York, 1964), pp. 138–159.

Biotin content of foods
in mcg per 100 g

* *best sources*	
wheat bran	14
wholewheat flour	7
wholewheat bread	6
* raw oatmeal	20
sponge cake without fat	15
dried skimmed milk	16
Camembert type cheese	6
cooked egg	25
fried kidney	42 – 53
* fried calf liver	53
* fried chicken liver	170
* fried lamb's liver	41
* stewed ox liver	50
stewed pig's liver	34
fried herring	10
fried cod's roe	15
avocado pear	3.2
tomato purée	8.0
dried yeast	200

Although raw egg yolk has a high level of biotin (60 mg per 100 g), it binds with the avidin in the white in such a way that man cannot digest it. However, if the white and yolk are both cooked, the avidin becomes inactive and the biotin can be absorbed. Poor sources of this vitamin are most meat and fish, vegetables and fruit and nuts. For a high biotin breakfast try a muesli made with raw oats and reconstituted dried skimmed milk plus an extra amount of granules, followed by a cooked egg on wholewheat toast. Non-vegetarians will benefit from homemade chicken liver pâté, which is very high in this vitamin. Although dried yeast has a very high level it is not eaten in very large amounts.

■Vitamin K

Vitamin K is found in many forms. Phytomenadione is the natural form vitamin K1. The form menaquinone, known as vitamin K2, is formed by bacterial action in a healthy intestine. Synthetic forms include acetomenaphthone, which is not as biologically potent as the natural forms, K1 and K2.

□*Oil-soluble.*

□*Natural sources* Green vegetables, yoghurt.

□*Main functions* A blood clotting agent.

□*Main deficiency symptoms* Nosebleeds, frequent haemorrhaging, miscarriages. If antibiotics have been taken, the friendly intestinal flora which produce vitamin K will be killed and so deficiency may result.

□*Co-factors* None.

□*Stability* Very stable, not significantly lost in cooking.

□*Overdosing and toxicity* Because vitamin K is biologically active in blood clotting processes, care should be taken in using pure supplements routinely, especially for people on a modern western diet where thrombosis is already a major killer. We are not aware of any pure supplements being available except on doctor's prescription. Vitamin K may be used by doctors to overcome problems associated with anti-coagulant drugs which may overthin the blood in some patients. Too much vitamin K would cause severe problems of thrombosis. It should only be used as a supplement in compound multivitamins, and the dose per day should not exceed 500 mcg.

□*RDA* 100 to 250 mcg.

■Vitamin P/Bioflavonoids, Hesperidin, Rutin & Troxerutin

□*Water-soluble.*

□*Natural sources* Buck wheat (rutin), peel of citrus fruits and rose hips (hesperidin).

□*Commercial forms for supplements* Various extracts are available with varying ratios of ingredient compositions. The purer the extract is in hesperidin or rutin, the better it is said to be nutritionally. The term bioflavonoids is meaningless as regards potency unless a reference to basic rutin or hesperidin content is stated.

□*Main functions* As strengtheners of blood vessels, especially the tiny capillaries in the skin. Broken vessels on the cheeks leading to unsightly red areas can sometimes be cleared using bioflavonoids. Rutin has been used by herbalists as a specific aid for lowering blood pressure.

□*Deficiency symptoms* Weakness of blood vessels, broken veins in the skin, susceptibility to infections.

□*Co-factors* Vitamin C – during colds and flu equal quantities of bioflavonoids and C are given; for protection the ratio of 1:10 (bioflavonoids to vitamin C) is often recommended.

□*Stability* Very stable, no losses in cooking.

□*Overdosing and toxicity* Not known.

□*RDA* Not officially a vitamin, but for general supplemental purposes take one tenth as much as vitamin C. Treatment for weak blood capillaries up to 1000 mg pure hesperidin daily for 4 to 6 weeks.

■Vitamin L

Ortho amino benzoic acid has been referred to as vitamin L1, whilst vitamin L2 is a much more complex substance. They are thought to be necessary for lactation but their dietary sources are not specified. Not generally recognized as vitamins.

■Vitamin T

A complex growth factor originally isolated from termites. Also claimed to be found in yeasts and fungi. No satisfactory structure has been proposed. Certainly not generally recognized as a vitamin.

■Vitamin X

A distinctly mythical substance found in a mysterious herbal mixture call fo-ti-tieng. This substance does not appear to have a single identity, but different herbs are sold for it in the UK and USA. A Chinese herbalist attributed his life span of 250 years to the herb. It appears that others then proposed the presence of a vitamin X as the long life giving factor. Perhaps this lead could prove an interesting research area for a young enthusiast.

■Vitamin U

Whilst some researchers have identified this as DL-methoinine-methylsulphonium chloride this is not accepted generally and no vitamin U exists as a single entity. It was the ulcer-preventive properties of certain fresh green vegetables which led to the proposal of a vitamin in them. These juices were found to be rich in vitamin C and the other components are difficult to identify because of general instability of the juices.

■7 Minerals

■Boron

This is an essential element for plants but there is no acceptable evidence of a human requirement. It occurs widely in plants but if they are grown on boron-deficient soils their growth is affected, e.g. pitted apples are a result of boron deficiency. Plant boron is ingested by humans but is excreted efficiently. Claims have been made that people living in boron-deficient areas suffer from more arthritic disease than others. Only anecdotal evidence exists and no scientific trials have supported this proposition. Most countries ban use of boron compounds like borax (sodium perborate) in over the counter drugs because of toxicity problems. Children have died as a result of accidental ingestion of doses exceeding 10 g. Supplementary amounts of boron recommended to help arthritis are some 200 times less than the toxic level. This is not an unusual relationship between an essential daily requirement of a nutrient and its toxicity, so perhaps boron will soon be seen in food supplement form.

■Bromine

Considered as a toxic substance both as bromine itself and as bromide, the form normally found in plants and seawater. Bromides were used as sleeping drugs before the discovery of barbiturates. Trace amounts of bromine may well be essential for metabolism but this is unproved. It is present widely in food and one may take in as much as 7.5 mg daily. No supplemental sources of pure bromite salts are available. It will be present in most dried vegetable products, such as kelp or alfalfa.

■Calcium

□*Natural sources*   Milk, cheese, cereals, fish, bones, dried apricots.

□*Commercial sources for supplements*   Bone meal, dolomite, various inorganic salts, such as calcium carbonate (chalk), calcium phosphate and calcium sulphate (plaster of paris). Organic salts, such as calcium lactate and gluconate, are better absorbed. Chalk is the normal starting material for the production of commercial calcium salts.

□*Main functions*   Calcium is the most abundant mineral in the body. Formation of bones and teeth. An important body electrolyte (as Ca^{++}) which is involved in blood clotting, nerve and muscle control, and heart condition. Often used as a co-factor as an aid to sleeping (the calcium content of milk is probably the element which makes that beverage an ideal bedtime drink).

□*Deficiency symptoms*   Brittle bones (rickets), insomnia, muscle cramps, heart palpitations, brittle fingernails (see Appendix).

□*Main co-factors*   Vitamin D, magnesium, phosphorus.

□*Overdosing and toxicity*   Mild constipation; alkalosis when the blood becomes too alkaline, but this is very rare since balanced salts are always used in nutritional supplements.

□*RDA*   500 mg of elemental calcium. Nutritionists sometimes recommend up to 2000 mg of elemental calcium.

□*Stability*   Calcium salts are very stable.

Calcium content of foods
in mg per 100 g

* best sources

wholewheat flour	35
white flour	150
white SR flour	350
raw oatmeal	55
low fat soya flour	240
rice	4
white bread	100
wholewheat bread	23
* muesli	200
rock cakes	390
shortcrust pastry	110

bread and butter pudding	130
milk pudding	130
* dried skimmed milk	1190
fresh milk	120
cottage cheese	60
* Cheddar cheese	800
* Parmesan	1220
* yoghurt	180
eggs	52
butter	15
margarine	4
fried cod	80
* fried haddock	110
plaice fried in crumbs	67
* canned pilchards	300
* sardines	550
* sprats	620
* whitebait	860
* shrimps	320
mussels	200
fish paste	280
boiled haricot beans	65
boiled broccoli tops	76
raw red cabbage	53
old raw carrots	48
mustard and cress	66
raw spring onion	140
raw parsley	330
* boiled spinach	600
* watercress	220
dried raw apricots	92
currants	95
dried figs	280
dates	68
whole lemons	110
stewed rhubarb	84
* almonds	250
brazils	180
black treacle	500
marzipan	120
* milk chocolate	220
cocoa powder	130
instant coffee	160

curry powder	640
mustard powder	330
yeast extract spread	95

From this list it can be seen that fruit and meat are poor sources. White flour has a higher level of calcium than wholewheat flour (and bread) because calcium is added during manufacture. Milk products and fish probably contribute most to the diet in the way of calcium as they can be eaten in quite large amounts, especially fish. Spinach is an extra good source but this is not the most popular of vegetables.

■Chlorine

This element in the chloride form provides an important balance in the body's electrolytes (as Cl). Many mineral elements, such as sodium and potassium, are balanced by chlorine in the form of sodium and potassium chlorides. In the form of chlorine gas it is toxic, although in low concentrations it is used to purify swimming pool water.

□*Natural sources*   Most food contains mineral chlorides, and chlorine is one of the world's most abundant elements.

□*Commercial sources for supplement*   Sodium chloride, potassium chloride, betaine hydrochloride.

□*Main functions*   An essential electrolyte component found throughout body tissues.

□*Deficiency symptoms*   Because it is closely associated with sodium, potassium and other minerals, its deficiency would be accompanied by their deficiency, leading to very serious health problems.

□*Main co-factors*   Minerals.

□*Overdosing and toxicity*   Its association with minerals makes its toxicity allied to theirs. It would be virtually impossible to get toxicity with just chloride – it must have partners. Free chlorine, such as is found in swimming pools and tap waters, destroys some vitamins, e.g. vitamin E, and may also kill friendly intestinal bacteria. Use of acidophilus supplements or consumption of fresh yoghurt counteracts the latter.

□*Stability*   Mineral chlorides are very stable.

□*RDA*   4 to 5 g.

■Chromium

□*Natural sources*   Whole wheat, whole grains, brewer's yeast, molasses.

□*Commercial sources for supplements*   High chromium yeast, chromium salts including chloride, orotate, gluconate and amino acid chelates.

□*Main function*   In carbohydrate metabolism. It forms part of the glucose tolerance factor essential in regulating blood sugar levels. Appears to be a factor in protecting from high cholesterol levels and development of arterial plaques which in turn lead to coronary heart disease.

□*Deficiency symptoms*   Heart and circulatory problems, glucose intolerance in diabetes.

□*Co-factors*   Polyunsaturated fatty acids.

□*Overdosing and toxicity*   Chromium is normally only taken in very small doses and in the chromic (Cr^{+++}) form. It is poorly absorbed from supplemental forms like the chloride but the organic salts (orotates, gluconates, amino acid chelates) are claimed to yield better blood levels. Supplements containing 10–20 mg of chromium salt (in the chromic form containing up to 5 mg elemental chromium) are quite safe. Chromium in valencies other than 3 should not be taken as a food supplement.

□*RDA*   Up to 200 mcg daily, but in supplements much more is often present because of poor absorption levels.

□*Stability*   Chromium salts are stable.

■Cobalt

□*Natural sources*   Occurs widely in trace amounts in foods. Animals can convert it to vitamin B12 and so animal-based foods provide the best essential source of the mineral.

□*Commercial sources for supplements*   Vitamin B12. Cobalt salts are often added to animal feed to ensure that they produce adequate vitamin B12 in their tissues.

□*Main functions*   Production of vitamin B12. May be linked with iodine in the formation of thyroid hormones.

□*Deficiency symptoms*   See vitamin B12 (page 80).

□*Co-factors*   Iodine.

□*Overdosing and toxicity* Cobalt occurs in minute traces in foodstuffs and food supplements. For human consumption, use only vitamin B12 as its source. The body readily excretes cobalt, so there is no danger of overdosing in normal circumstances.

□*RDA* See vitamin B12.

■Copper

□*Natural sources* Oysters and shellfish, liver, legumes, nuts and raisins.

□*Commercial sources for supplements* Copper sulphate, orotate, gluconate, amino acid chelates.

□*Main functions* Bone, red blood cell and haemoglobin formation, associated with many enzyme systems involved in emotional states and mental processes. May have a relevance in cancer prevention. Hair colour and skin condition require adequate amounts of copper.

□*Deficiency symptoms* Skin lesions, general weakness, diarrhoea in infants.

□*Co-factors* Vitamin A, zinc and iron, vitamin C.

□*Overdosing and toxicity* Copper is seldom found in supplements on its own but is present in most general multimineral mixtures. Large doses of copper sulphate, the most economical commercial source of copper, will cause vomiting. It is therefore difficult to achieve toxic blood levels.

□*RDA* 2–3 mg daily as elemental copper equivalent to approximately 10 mg dried copper sulphate.

□*Stability* Copper salts are very stable.

Copper content of foods
in mg per 100 g

* best sources

wheat bran	1.34
wheat germ	1.20
All-Bran	1.2
Puffed Wheat	0.56
Weetabix	0.54
* fried calf liver	12.0

fried chicken liver	0.53
*fried lamb's liver	9.9
stewed ox liver	2.3
stewed pig's liver	2.5
*crab	4.8
lobster	1.7
shrimps	0.8
raw oysters	0.9
raw mushrooms	0.64
fried mushrooms	0.78
raw parsley	0.52
currants	0.48
raw, dried peaches	0.63
brazil nuts	0.50
dessicated coconut	0.55
smooth peanut butter	0.70
glacé cherries	1.28
plain chocolate	0.70
cocoa powder	3.9
drinking chocolate	1.1
tomato purée	0.63
pepper	1.13
yeast (dried)	5.0

Milk and milk products, fruit and vegetables are poor sources of copper and so is fish. Best sources for vegetarians and vegans are wheat germ, brazil nuts and mushrooms.

■Fluorine

□*Natural sources* In various mineral ores, mainly in association with calcium. Present in seawater as sodium fluoride.

□*Commercial sources for supplements* Sodium fluoride, calcium fluoride, bone meal.

□*Main functions* Resistance to tooth decay.

□*Deficiency symptoms* Tooth decay.

□*Overdosing and toxicity* Sodium fluoride is added to drinking water in some areas at a level to provide one part fluorine to a million parts water. This is below the level in seawater whence all life emanates, and also below the natural levels found in drinking water in many countries. Amounts not far in excess of those in seawater can be harmful and this is one of the reasons why such controversy rages about adding sodium fluoride to drinking water. Another reason is that people object to mass medication when only children benefit whilst others may be harmed. The over-boiling of artificially fluoridated water will cause concentration of the fluoride which may also cause health problems. Whilst one part per million protects against tooth decay in children, 2 to 3 parts per million cause tooth discolouration and ten parts per million may cause bone damage.

□*RDA*   Less than 0.1 mg.

■Iodine

Iodine is the heaviest of the four halogen elements. Fluorine, chlorine and bromine are the other halogens.

□*Natural sources*   Seafood, kelp (seaweed), thyroid gland.

□*Commercial sources for supplements*   Seaweed, potassium iodide, dried thyroid (hormone free).

□*Main functions*   Iodine is an essential element in the formation of thyroid hormones. These hormones control the speed of many metabolic processes, especially fat burning and energy production.

□*Deficiency symptoms*   Goitre – a swelling in the neck where the thyroid gland is situated. This condition was known as Derbyshire neck as people in Derbyshire had diets very low in natural iodine and goitres were very common. The addition of iodine to drinking water and salt (iodized salt) is a preventative against goitre. Symptoms of cold hands and feet, rapid fatigue and overweight are associated with deficiency.

□*Overdosing and toxicity*   Like other halogens, excesses of iodine are toxic to metabolic processes. Free iodine, which is a powerful antiseptic, is never used in foods. It is the inorganic iodide and bound organic forms which are used. The normal form of supplementation is wild sea kelp. Sometimes kelp tablets are boosted with potassium or sodium iodide to provide a guaranteed iodine content. It is not advisable for anyone to take more than 500 mcg of free iodine supplementally for a prolonged period, but natural iodine from organic sources such as kelp has no known toxicity levels and 3 to 6 tablets with as much as 200 mcg organic iodine each are often used supplementally.

□*RDA*   150 to 200 mcg as free iodine.

■Iron

There are two basic natural irons: ferrous and ferric. In Latin nomenclature the term 'Ferri' is often used and confusingly this refers to ferrous iron, which is the nutritionally active form.

□*Natural sources*   Haemoglobin and dried blood, meat, poultry, cereals, seafood, black-strap molasses, liver.

□*Commercial sources for supplements*   Ferrous irons salts, especially sulphate, fumarate, gluconate, orotate, proteinate/amino acid chelates. Liver and dried haemoglobin. Iron is better absorbed in the presence of vitamin C because this ensures that it is in the ferrous form.

□*Main functions*   Haemoglobin production, which is vital to the oxygen-carrying capacity of blood. Growth in children and stress situations.

□*Deficiency symptoms*   Classical anaemia (non iron deficiency anaemias should not be treated with iron salts), showing pale skin and fatigue. Severe blood losses will lead to deficiencies, e.g. in menstruating women. Brittle finger nails and breathlessness.

□*Co-factors*   Vitamin C, vitamin B12 and folic acid, copper, manganese, glutathione.

□*Overdosing and toxicity*   The body rejects excess iron fairly easily and only some 5 to 10% taken in food is absorbed. Too much iron in supplemental form will cause severe constipation. Some iron salts cause gastric irritation in some people and this is related to the relative iron concentration. Iron gluconate, fumarate and orotate are said not to produce so much gastric irritation as the sulphate and are therefore better sources of nutritional iron. Substained release products are formulated to protect against gastric side effects. Daily intakes of more than 100 mg elemental iron are inadvisable except under professional direction. This problem of gastric irritation increasing with mineral concentration within compounds is found with many other minerals, e.g. copper, zinc, manganese, chromium.

□*RDA*   10 to 15 mg, but only 1 to 2 mg of this is absorbed. A sensible supplemental level would be 15 to 20 mg elemental ferrous iron daily.

□*Stability*   Iron is better absorbed in the ferrous form but this is less stable than the ferric form. Formulation of supplements with ascorbic acid (vitamin C) ensures greater stability of ferrous iron compounds.

Iron content of foods
in mg per 100 g

* *best sources*

* wheat germ	10.0
wheat bran	12.9
wholewheat flour	4.0
raw oatmeal	4.1
low fat soya flour	9.1
* bread with wheat germ	4.5
malt bread	3.6
white bread	1.7
wholewheat bread	2.5
* All-Bran	12.0
* Special K	20.0
Shredded Wheat	4.2
* Weetabix	7.6
rye crispbread	3.7
oatcakes	4.5
eggs	2.0
lean, grilled steak	3.4
lean leg of lamb	2.7
lean leg of pork	1.3
dark chicken meat	1.9
light chicken meat	0.6
lean roast duck	2.7
* grouse	7.6
* partridge	7.7
* pheasant	8.4
* roast pigeon	19.4
dark turkey meat	1.2
* stewed hare	10.8
* venison	7.8
stewed ox heart	7.7
* fried lamb's kidney	12.0
* fried calf liver	9.5
* chicken liver	9.4
* stewed ox liver	7.8
* stewed pig's liver	17.0
corned beef	2.9
* black pudding	20.0
fried beefburgers	3.1
baked cod	0.4
fried haddock	1.2

grilled herring	1.0
sardines	2.4
fried sprats	4.5
*cockles	26.0
*mussels	7.7
raw oysters	6.0
fish paste	9.0
boiled butter beans	1.7
*boiled haricot beans	2.5
boiled broccoli tops	1.0
boiled leeks	2.0
cooked lentils	2.4
lettuce	0.9
raw mushrooms	1.0
fried mushrooms	1.3
mustard and cress	1.0
spring onions	1.2
raw parsley	8.0
peas	1.2
canned processed peas	1.5
cooked dried peas	1.4
cooked dried split peas	1.7
jacket potatoes	0.6
chips	0.9
roast potatoes	0.7
boiled spring greens	1.3
boiled swede	1.1
boiled turnip tops	3.1
fresh raw apricots	0.4
raw dried apricots	4.1
avocado pears	1.5
stewed blackcurrants	1.0
currants	1.8
dried raw figs	4.2
stewed figs (dried)	2.2
dates	1.6
loganberries	1.4
dried raw peaches	6.8
dried raw prunes	2.9
stewed prunes	1.4
raisins	1.6

raspberries	1.2
sultanas	1.8
* almonds	4.2
brazils	2.8
hazel nuts	1.1
peanuts	2.0
walnuts	2.4
black treacle	9.2
milk chocolate	1.6
plain chocolate	2.4
cocoa powder	10.5
instant coffee	4.4
drinking chocolate	2.4
white wine (dry)	0.5
white wine (medium)	1.21
red wine	0.9
rosé wine	0.95
tomato purée	5.1
sweet pickle	2.0
curry powder	75.0
ground ginger	17.2
mustard powder	10.9
pepper	10.2
vinegar	5.0
yeast	20.0

You will see from this list that the darker meats contain much higher levels of iron than lighter meats. Although some items seem very high in iron they are only eaten in small amounts, e.g. curry powder and parsley. Some foods which are lower in iron content are in fact more useful as a source because they can be eaten in quite large amounts, e.g. haricot beans. Game meats have very good levels of iron, while milk, dairy products, fats and oils are very poor sources in the diet. In dried fruits the concentration of iron is higher than for the fresh versions. The level goes down when the fruit is soaked in water, but larger quantities of soaked fruit can be eaten than dried, which evens things out. High iron level can be expected in breakfast cereals because they are fortified with extra iron during processing.

■Magnesium

□*Natural sources*   Green vegetables, cereals, bone meal, honey, kelp and chlorophyll.

□*Commercial sources for suppplements* Dolomite, magnesium carbonate, magnesium oxide or hydroxide, magnesium orotate and amino acid chelates, chlorophyll.

□*Main functions*   It is a very important mineral in cell function and a co-factor in numerous enzyme systems. Muscular and nervous control systems depend upon it. It is also thought to be important in stabilizing fundamental nucleic acid structures (RNA/DNA). It plays a part in bone and tooth formation as well as heart and circulation health.

□*Deficiency symptoms* Nervousness, tremors, rapid pulse, confusion and disorientation, hyperactivity, heart beat irregularity and heart arrest.

□*Co-factors*   Calcium, phosphorus, vitamin B6.

□*Overdosing and toxicity*   On a normal regime of supplementation there are no dangers. Long-term high doses of antacids or laxatives containing magnesium salts may give problems. Excessive magnesium (over 20 g daily) may lead to low blood pressure, heart problems, drowsiness, thirst and coma.

□*RDA*   200 – 500 mg daily, but supplemental levels up to 1000 mg are often recommended by nutritionists usually in balance with calcium. Magnesium is not particularly efficiently absorbed from food and people with general malabsorption problems may well need to use large supplemental doses to achieve adequate blood levels and body stores. More is needed in pregnancy and lactation.

□*Stability*   Magnesium salts are very stable.

Magnesium content of foods
in mg per 100 g

* *best sources*

* wheat bran	520
wheat germ	300
* wholewheat flour	140
white flour	36
raw oatmeal	110
* low fat soya flour	290

rye flour	92
All-Bran	370
muesli	100
Puffed Wheat	140
Shredded Wheat	130
dried, skimmed milk	117
*shrimps	110
winkles	360
raw parsley	52
boiled spinach	59
dried, raw apricots	65
dried, raw figs	92
dates	59
*almonds	260
*brazils	410
fresh peanuts	180
walnuts	130
black treacle	140
marzipan	120
cocoa powder	520
salt	140
mustard powder	260
instant coffee	390
yeast extract spread	180
curry powder	280

Several foods with high levels of magnesium cannot be considered as good sources as they are only eaten in very small amounts: e.g. 100 g of mustard powder would probably not be consumed by one person in a whole year. Although winkles have a high level, how many people are able to buy them or would favour eating them?

■Manganese

□*Natural sources*   Cereals, green leafy vegetables, nuts, legumes and celery.

□*Commercial sources for supplements*   Manganese sulphate, gluconate, orotate and amino acid chelates.

□*Main functions*   Various enzyme systems involved in reproductive processes and sex hormone formation. Fat and carbohydrate metabolism. Vitamin B1 metabolism. Memory and irritability are nerve conditions depending in part on this mineral.

□*Deficiency symptoms*   None officially recognized, but some nutritionists have postulated deafness and ear noises as possibly related to manganese deficiency.

□*Co-factors*   Biotin, vitamin B, and vitamin C.

□*Overdosing and toxicity*   Usually only used in multimineral supplements in very small amounts and there is no danger of toxicity in normal circumstances. Single dose supplements, even if they provide substantial amounts of manganese of up to 20 mg, are unlikely to cause problems because absorption into the blood stream is not very efficient.

□*RDA*   2–3 mg. Supplements containing 10 mg of elemental manganese are sometimes used.

□*Stability*   Manganese salts are very stable.

■Molybdenum

□*Natural sources*   Cereals, yeast, green vegetables, legumes.

□*Commercial sources for supplements*   Sodium or potassium molybdate, high molybdenum yeast.

□*Main functions*   In enzyme systems, especially the conversion of purines (for example caffeine) to uric acid. Detoxifies the aldehydes which collect in body processes. Legumes contain purines and provide molybdenum too so that this aids their metabolism.

□*Deficiency symptoms*   Nothing specific and molybdenum may not be an essential mineral. It prevents tooth decay in rats.

□*Co-factors*   There is some evidence of inter-action with copper and iron.

□*Overdosing and toxicity*   Molybdenum is only used supplementarily in minute amounts of about 100 mcg and requirements are not thought to exceed this. Excessive intake has been linked to gout because of the part that the mineral plays in the enzyme systems which convert purines to uric acid. This evidence is not conclusive.

□*RDA*   100 mcg, or 2 mcg per kilogram of body weight.

□*Stability*   Molybdenum compounds used in supplements are very stable.

■Phosphorus

This element is found in various combined forms both with inorganic minerals, e.g. as phosphates of calcium or iron, and in organic compounds such as phosphatides in lecithin. In the form of yellow phosphorus it is highly dangerous and will catch fire in air. Red and black phosphoruses are not so dangerous but have no use in nutrition.

□*Natural sources* It is found in all foods in the combined phosphate or phosphatide form. Eggs, meat, poultry, milk, grains, fish and legumes are all sources.

□*Commercial sources for supplements* Calcium phosphates, bone meal and lecithin.

□*Main functions* Forms vital phosphate linkages found throughout body structures and general metabolic systems.

□*Deficiency* Would have serious consequences for body processes in general.

□*Main co-factors* Calcium, iron, vitamin D and polyunsaturates.

□*Overdosing and toxicity* No toxicity in the forms found in foods and supplements.

□*RDA* 800 to 1200 mg.

□*Stability* Phosphates are very stable.

■Potassium

□*Natural sources* Green vegetables, fresh fruit, dried fruit, nuts, seafood, sunflower seeds, legumes.

□*Commercial sources for supplements* Potassium salts, especially chloride, bicarbonate, gluconate and orotate.

□*Main functions* Heart and blood circulation, muscle function. Potassium is involved in many body processes and is the principal mineral in intracellular fluid. It is essential for carbohydrate metabolism and energy production, glycogen storage (i.e. energy stores) and protein metabolism. It is closely associated with sodium and is excreted in preference to that mineral by the kidney.

□*Deficiency symptoms* Very severe because of potassium's wide occurrence in intracellular fluid as a balancing electrolyte.

Thirst, dry skin, irregular heart beat, loss of reflexes, nervousness, insomnia, muscle weakness, vomiting, mental confusion, respiratory failure and heart problems.

□*Co-factors*   Sodium and vitamin B6.

□*Overdosing and toxicity*   Generally non toxic, but supplement tablets formulated with potassium chloride may cause ulceration and irritation to stomach and intestinal linings owing to localized overconcentration as the tablet bolus breaks down.

A potassium chloride supplement should be used in solution or as a crystalline powder such as a salt substitute where no localized over-concentration can take place. Other salts of potassium, such as the bicarbonate or orotate, do not appear to give the same problems. People taking diuretics which chemically interfere with kidney function to conserve potassium should not use potassium supplements and should watch their intake of potassium rich foods. People with renal insufficiency or suffering from heat cramp and severe dehydration should not be given potassium supplements without medical supervision.

□*RDA*   Approximately 4000 mg. Potassium is readily absorbed from food, but excess is also rapidly excreted in urine. Supplements usually provide about 1000 to 2000 mg daily. The body contains some 120 g of potassium.

□*Stability*   Potassium salts are very stable.

□*High potassium food*

Here, for one person, is a main meal that is high in potassium and low in sodium. It comprises cold meat, salad and hot potato followed by fruit. It should be prepared just before eating so that the raw vegetables do not deteriorate. Dress the salad with a little oil/vinegar dressing – one part vinegar to 2 parts oil (sunflower).

Salad: 1 oz (100 g) each of raw sliced mushrooms, shredded red or white cabbage and cooked butterbeans. Sprinkle with a little freshly chopped parsley and a few raisins and toss in a little dressing. Season with just black pepper, freshly ground. Eat with 2 oz (50 g) cold roast beef, trimmed of fat, 2 tomatoes and a jacket potato with a small knob of polyunsaturated margarine. (Over 1,150 mg potassium.)

Dessert: Wash 2 oz (50 g) dried apricots. Soak overnight in cold water. The following day cook in the soaking water for about 20 to 30 minutes, until tender. Use a saucepan and top it up with water if necessary. Add a little brown sugar or honey if the fruit is too sharp. (A 4 oz (100 g) portion of the cooked apricots plus the juice has a potassium value of over 650 mg.) For full potassium value this meal should not have salt added. Total meal has over 1,800 mg potassium.

Bread and potassium

The average baker's wholewheat loaf contains approximately 220 mg of potassium per 100 g and only 100 mg in the same amount of white bread. As both types of bread are likely to contain about 540 mg of sodium per 100 g, this really cancels out the potassium value. By making your own bread at home, leaving out the salt, and boosting the wholewheat flour with wheat germ, soya and wheat bran, the potassium value of your bread can be increased considerably. This type of bread would be helpful to people who do not get enough potassium from their vegetables, such as those who eat snack lunches at work. The bread can be used in sandwiches, and fresh fruit can be used as an accompaniment to boost further the potassium level of a snack meal. Here are some helpful figures:

Food	potassium	sodium
	approx mg per 100 g (4 oz)	
baker's wholewheat bread	220	540
baker's white bread	100	540
rye crispbread	500	220
wheat germ	1000	4
wheat bran	1160	28
soya flour (low fat)	2030	1
wholewheat flour	360	3
white flour	130	3

Two foods used as starters are high in potassium and low in sodium:

asparagus (cooked)	240	2
avocado (raw)	400	2

Breakfast, normally a low potassium meal for most people, can be boosted with fruit juice or fruit, and if a cooked course is served, mushrooms can be added:

grapefruit juice	110	3
pineapple juice	140	1
fried mushrooms	570	11

High protein foods are usually high in sodium too. Here are four with the least sodium:

lean grilled rumpsteak	380	55
roast grouse	470	96
grilled herring	370	170
fried mackerel	420	150

While vegetables are always considered to be a good source of potassium in the diet because they are eaten in quite large quantities, poor cooking can result in potassium losses. Raw vegetables are the best source and this is why salads are so important a part of our food:

raw white cabbage	390	7
raw red cabbage	300	32
cauliflower (raw)	350	8
mushrooms (raw)	470	9
lettuce	240	9
tomatoes	290	3

Potatoes have a high potassium level and can be eaten in large amounts. Different methods of cooking offer different levels:

jacket potatoes (eaten with skins)	550	6
chips	1020	12
new potatoes (boiled)	330	41
roast potatoes	750	9

When cooking green vegetables, steaming and using the water from the steaming that is left in the saucepan (if any) to make the gravy ensures only a small loss of potassium:

Brussels sprouts	240	2
spinach	490	120

Some foods have a very high potassium level but as they are only eaten in very small amounts their value in the diet is not high:

instant coffee	1000	41
Indian tea	2160	45
dried yeast	2000	50
tomato purée	1540	20
parsley (fresh raw)	1080	33

Most fresh fruits have good potassium levels if they are eaten raw. They are also low in sodium and can be eaten in quite large quantities. The fruits with highest levels are listed here:

bananas	350	1
cherries	310	4
apricots	320	trace
grapes	320	2

One excellent source of potassium is butterbeans (cooked):

butterbeans	400	16

Dried fruits, although lacking in vitamins through drying, have high concentrations of potassium as a result. Use raw in salads as well as in baking:

currants	710	20
dried figs	1010	87
dates (stoned)	750	5
dried peaches (raw)	1100	6
prunes, dried stoned	860	12
raisins	860	52
sultanas	860	53
peaches, dried raw	1100	6
apricots, dried raw	1880	56

Nuts are both high in potassium and low in sodium. The amounts given are for nuts weighed in their shells. Figures are estimated on the edible kernels obtained from 100 g of nuts in shell:

almonds	860	6
brazils	760	2
chestnuts	500	11
walnuts	630	3

A combination of dried fruit and nuts makes an excellent high potassium snack.
Miscellaneous information of interest:

white sugar	2	*trace*
black treacle	1470	96
sweet sherry	110	13

The basic point to remember about potassium high foods is that the presence of a high level of sodium detracts from the potassium value. Best value is from foods which are high in potassium and low in sodium.

High potassium fruit cake

A wholefood cake with a mixture of high potassium dried fruits.

Ingredients ½ lb (225 g) wholewheat flour, 1 heaped teaspoon baking powder, 1 level teaspoon each of mixed spice and cinnamon, 5 oz (140 g) polyunsaturated margarine, 4 oz (100 g) brown sugar, 3 eggs (beaten), a little milk to mix, 4 oz (100 g) each of currants, stoned dates (chopped), stoned prunes (chopped), dried apple rings (chopped) and dried pears (chopped), the grated rind of 1 lemon and 1 orange.

Method Preheat oven at Gas Mark 4 (350°F/180°C). Grease and flour an 8" (20 cm) cake tin. Put the flour into a mixing bowl and sprinkle in the baking powder and spices. Mix well. Add the margarine, sugar and eggs. Mix, then beat, adding a little milk to make a mixture that will drop slowly from the spoon. Stir in the dried fruit and rinds. Bake on the middle shelf for about 2 hours, turning the oven down slightly after the first half hour. Let the cake cool in the tin for a few minutes so that it shrinks away from the sides. Turn out carefully on to a wire rack and allow to grow cold. Store in an airtight tin.

Even more potassium can be added to this cake by decorating the top of the cake, before baking, with shelled almonds. However, this also adds more fat to the recipe.

■Selenium

□*Natural sources* Whole cereals, seafoods, meat, eggs, brewer's yeast.

□*Commercial sources for supplements* Special high selenium yeasts, where the yeast has been grown on a medium rich in selenium and has bound it chemically into the protein structure. The industrial chemicals sodium selenite and sodium selenate have been used but are, in our opinion, not suitable for dietary purposes. Their attraction to manufacturers for supplements is their cheapness – approximately 100 times cheaper than genuine organically bound selenium.

□*Main functions* It acts with free radical scavengers like vitamin E together with protectors like vitamin A to prolong cell life. It is claimed to have a protective part to play in fighting degenerative diseases including cancer and arthritis. Men may need more selenium than women – it is lost in semen and concentrated in the male genital glands.

□*Deficiency symptoms* It has been shown that populations living in areas of the USA where selenium in the soil is low have greater susceptibility to cancer. Premature aging pigmentation is another deficiency symptom. In animals, still-births and wasting of young may be prevented by adding selenium to the diet where the soil is deficient in that mineral. Liver and skin diseases are also reported to be greater in animals grazing on selenium-deficient soil.

□*Co-factors* Vitamin E, glutathione, vitamin C and A or be-tacarotene.

□*Overdosing and toxicity*   We do not advise taking more than 200 mcg daily in supplemental form. It should be taken in the organic form. Supplements prepared using sodium selenite and selenate will contain variable levels of selenium. One individual tablet could contain 50% more than the label claims yet the average content of 100 tablets would equal that claim. Inherent manufacturing problems with low dose substances are responsible for this variation. Recently a company in the USA prepared selenium tablets which contained no less than 150 mg instead of 150 mcg, an error which could only have occurred if sodium selenite instead of the organically bound selenium on yeast had been used. Always check the labels of selenium supplement aids carefully. Yeast grown and 'yeast absorbed' are different. Some companies have already tried to fool consumers by just adding sodium selenite to dried brewer's yeast. This is just a mixture made by adding sodium selenite to dead yeast – the selenium you would ingest would be that derived from the sodium selenite not from yeast. Yeast-bound selenium is prepared on live yeasts which are killed only after the selenium has been built into their structure.

□*RDA*   150 to 200 mcg.

□*Stability*   Organically bound selenium in yeast is very stable.

■Silicon

This is the most abundant element on earth and is usually found in the form of silicon dioxide. Our bodies contain about 18 g of silicon in structural tissue.

□*Natural sources*   Herbs renowned for their tough stems and leaves, e.g. horsetail herb. Soluble mineral silicates like sodium silicate are found in sea water and traces in drinking water.

□*Commercial sources for supplements*   Dry horsetail herb is a rich source of organic silicon. Mineral silicates, such as sodium silicate. Silicon is frequently used as a natural additive in foods.

□*Main functions*   Many naturopaths believe that silicon and calcium are closely related in the body's metabolism. Weaknesses of bone and connective tissue (collagen) are particularly related to silicon status. Skin, nail and hair condition. Supplementary silicon may help speed the healing of bone fractures, wounds and burns.

□*Deficiency symptoms*   None recognized, but since silicon is an essential mineral, it is found particularly in skin and connective tissue. Slow healing of wounds and sprains might be considered evidence of deficiency of organic or absorbable silicon in the diet.

□*Co-factors*   Calcium.

□*Overdosing and toxicity*   None. Silicon is so poorly absorbed from food that practically all passes straight through the body.

□*RDA*   None.

□*Stability*   Silicon compounds are very stable.

■Silver

Not an essential mineral, but we are exposed to it in the form of eating utensils and through some industrial processes. Although traces may be found in our bodies through pollution, no toxic effects have been ascribed to it.

■Sodium

□*Natural sources*   Salt, sea salt, milk, cheese. Also found widely in convenience and processed foods as flavour enhancers and preservatives, e.g. in breads, cakes, cereals, biscuits, sausages.

□*Commercial sources of supplements*   Sodium chloride, sea salt.

□*Main functions*   Essential to life, but the body contains less sodium than potassium. It is the third most concentrated mineral electrolyte in the body. It is found in extra-cellular fluid, whereas potassium predominates in intra-cellular fluid. It is important for proper muscle contraction. It is lost in sweat and where people sweat greatly because of their jobs, e.g. blast-furnace workers and coal miners, it is advisable to use sodium replacements. Travellers moving from a cold to a warm climate without acclimatization may also need extra sodium.

□*Deficieny symptoms*   Heat stroke, fatigue, anorexia and many other symptoms, because absence of sodium will have an effect on many metabolic processes. Deficiency in the absence of excessive sweating is most unlikely with a normal diet.

□*Co-factors*   Potassium.

□*Overdosing and toxicity*   Sodium is naturally retained by the body to the exclusion of potassium. Modern diets with lots of processed foods containing sodium may be causing depletion of potassium.

Some researchers believe that we are consuming more than 20 times the amount of sodium needed daily for metabolism but too little potassium. It is probably not necessary to take any added salt. Excess salt leads to expansion of volume of extra-cellular fluid in the body, i.e. bloating. Correction of dietary sodium levels by elimination of the hidden sodium in processed foods often helps slimmers instantly as their bloating is reduced. Too much sodium in the diet has been implicated as one factor in high blood pressure, which leads to coronary heart disease and strokes. Sodium-restricted diets have been used to help kidney disease but are mainly used to bring high blood pressure back to normal.

□*RDA*   2000 to 3500 mg.

□*Stability*   Sodium salts are very stable.

Sodium content of foods
in mg per 100 g

plain flour	3
self-raising flour	350
raw oats	33
porridge	580
rice	6
pasta	5
bread	540 – 580
All-Bran	1670
cornflakes	1160
Shredded Wheat	8
Puffed Wheat	4
digestive biscuits	440
oatcakes	1230
water biscuits	470
rye crispbread	220
sponge cake	420
rich fruit cake	170
jam tarts	230
shortcrust pastry	480
scones	800
ice cream	70 – 80
milk pudding	53
treacle tart	360

You can see from this list that basic items such as rice and flour are very low in sodium. It is only when they are processed that the sodium content rises, sometimes quite drastically; e.g. self-raising flour contains a raising agent that is high in sodium, while plain flour does not. (This makes a difference of 347 mg per 100 g.) Traditionally salt is added to cooked oats making them quite high in sodium. It is surprising to see just how much sodium there is in sweet foods, e.g. biscuits, cake etc. Other foods which are considered to be bland, such as bread, have salt added to them to make them keep longer and this pushes up the level of sodium in what is basically a low sodium based flour product. Some breakfast cereals have salt added to them while others do not.

Sodium content of foods (contd)
in mg per 100 g

cow's milk	50
salted butter	870
single cream	42
cottage cheese	450
Cheddar cheese	610
Camembert type cheese	1410
yoghurt	64 – 76
eggs	140
scrambled eggs	1050
margarine	800
vegetable oils	*trace*
lean bacon	1870
lean beef	61
lean lamb	88
lean pork	370
lean chicken	72 – 80
brain	210
kidney	270 – 370
liver	76 – 130
corned beef	950
grilled pork sausages	1000
beefburgers	600
baked cod	340
fried haddock	180
smoked haddock	1220
plaice fried in crumbs	220

kippers	990
fresh salmon	110
smoked salmon	1880
sardines (canned)	680
canned tuna	420
prawns	1590
scampi	380
cockles	3520
fish fingers	320
fish paste	600

The salt added to some kinds of cheese during production accounts for the high level of sodium in the more solid kinds that still remain creamy, such as Brie or Camembert. Margarine and butter are salted to make them keep as well as taste good. Even unsalted butter still contains a little sodium. As bacon is preserved partly by salting, it has a high level of sodium. Salt is almost always added to meat during processing, especially pork products which go bad very quickly without it.

As you would expect, fish, etc. from salt water have a higher sodium content than those from fresh water. A good deal of salt is used in the manufacture of smoked fish.

■Sulphur

□*Natural sources*   Occurs widely in foods in the form of the sulphate radical (SO_4) and in proteins.

□*Commercial sources for supplements*   Sulphur-containing amino acids, e.g. methionine, cysteine. Mineral sulphates not well absorbed in that form.

□*Main functions*   As a mineral carrier and balancer in body tissues. The body contains about 140 g of sulphur. The sulphur-containing amino acids are usually involved in detoxifying processes.

□*Deficiency symptoms*   None known.

□*Co-factors*   Minerals.

□*Overdosing and toxicity*   None known for dietary sulphur.

□*RDA*   None.

□*Stability*   All dietary forms of sulphur are stable.

■Zinc

□*Natural sources*   Nuts, grains, legumes, oysters, seafoods, liver and meat.

□*Commercial sources for supplements*   Zinc oxide, sulphate, gluconate, orotate and amino acid chelates.

□*Main functions*   In many enzyme systems, including prostate gland function, protein metabolism, wound and burn healing, reproductive organ development, carbohydrate digestion.

□*Deficiency symptoms*   Retarded growth and anaemia, loss of taste, white spots on finger nails, prolonged wound healing, sterility, delayed sexual maturity.

□*Co-factors*   Vitamin B6, phosphorus, calcium.

□*Antifactor*   Excessive intake of cereal brans with high phytate content may deplete the zinc available to the body from food.

□*Overdosing and toxicity*   Large doses of zinc salts (600 mg) are emetic (make you sick). Simple inorganic salts like sulphate and chloride are the most potent in this regard – probably because they contain more zinc as a percentage than the organic salts like the gluconate. (See Iron, page 116).

□*RDA*   2 to 3 mg. Most supplemental regimes recommend 20 to 100 mg of elemental zinc daily in divided doses. Zinc gluconate contains about 15% zinc, so a 100 mg tablet yields only 15 mg zinc. Check that labels of supplements quote elemental zinc rather than the compound content, which will be considerably in excess of the actual zinc content.

□*Stability*   All zinc salts are very stable.

Zinc content of foods
in mg per 100 g

* *best sources*

* wheat bran	16.2
wholewheat bread	2.0
* All-Bran	8.4
Puffed Wheat	2.8
dried skimmed milk	4.1
Edam type cheese	4.0
Parmesan	4.0
eggs	1.5
grilled lean back rasher	3.7

* lean grilled steak	4.9
* lean roast beef	4.9
* roast leg of lamb (lean)	4.6
lean pork chop	3.5
light chicken meat	1.0
dark chicken meat	3.1
* fried calf liver	6.2
fried lamb's liver	4.0
* corned beef	5.6
fried beefburgers	4.2
sardines	3.0
* crab	5.5
* raw oysters	45.0
fresh peanuts	3.0
walnuts	3.0
hazelnuts	2.4
cocoa powder	6.9
ground ginger	6.8
dry mustard	6.5
* dried yeast	8.0

The star of this list is raw oysters, which contain a staggering amount of zinc. Fish is generally a poor source and so are fruit and vegetables.

■Gold

Although found in traces in body tissues, it is not considered essential as a nutrient. Gold based drug compounds have been used to treat rheumatoid arthritis and certain cancers. However, these treatments are not widely used.

■Lithium

Not proved as an essential mineral but found in traces in body tissues. It is present in seawater. A close relative of sodium and potassium. Used as a drug to help manic depressive disease. Lithium compounds should not be included in dietary supplements.

■Rubidium

Has been referred to as an essential mineral. It is assumed that only traces are required and would be obtained from foods. No pure rubidium supplements are available and little is known of this mineral's role in body metabolism.

■Germanium

Another mineral sometimes referred to as a nutrient, but no evidence of its role in nutrition exists. It is present in traces in the environment. No supplement necessary.

■Barium

Has been classified as essential, but only traces appear to be present in the body and foods. No nutritional role established. High doses of soluble barium salts are very toxic.

■Tin

There is no evidence that tin is essential for nutrition. It is found in traces in the body probably because of the use of tin in food canning.

■Aluminium

Not an essential mineral, but its content in the body has increased in recent times owing to the widespread use of aluminium cooking utensils and indigestion/antacid drugs based on aluminium compounds. There is some evidence to suggest that high levels of this mineral may be implicated in some degenerative illnesses, especially senile dementia. It would be a sensible health precaution to avoid unnecessary contact with this mineral, e.g. do not use aluminium cooking pans or aluminium based indigestion remedies.

■Strontium

A widely distributed mineral deposited in minute amounts in bones and teeth. Whether it is essential to these structures is debatable. No deficiency state has been found or toxic levels from pollution. It is the radioactive form strontium 90 from atomic bomb fall-out which presents the potentially serious health problem of leukaemia. Strontium 90 is absorbed into the bones where the white blood cells are made.

■Nickel

Not proved as an essential mineral for human nutrition, but is found in traces in plants and animals. May be essential for growth of a healthy foetus. It is present in supplements based on kelp or alfalfa. Supplementation in amounts exceeding 10 mcg not justified. Toxic in high doses.

■Vanadium

Normally referred to as an essential nutrient for man, but evidence is not widely accepted. Has been shown to be essential for the growth of rats. Only very small traces would be needed and these will normally be obtained in foods and supplements with herbal bases such as kelp or alfalfa. Sodium orthovanadate has been put into general mineral supplements at a concentration yielding about 10 mcg of vanadium. Toxic in high doses. It has been found to lower serum cholesterol in some humans but not generally.

■Arsenic

This element is from the same periodic group as phosphorus and it has been proposed as essential for life. We doubt this, but deficiency is impossible since it is contained in practically every food substance, and governments set strict limits on its permitted levels in substances for human consumption, including drugs.

As a matter of interest, in the days before modern acne preparations, doctors used to prescribe tin and tin oxide tablets for acne sufferers. In the 1950s the level of arsenic contamination allowed in these tablets was reduced dramatically and so were their effectiveness and sales. So perhaps here is some anecdotal evidence for arsenic's role in nutrition. Arsenic was used in the past as an important basis for anti-venereal disease drugs. The form used was quite different from the arsenic in the tin tablets.

■Titanium

Not an essential mineral, but is used widely in the form of titanium dioxide as a whitener for foodstuffs and drugs. In this form it is harmless.

■Tissue salts (biochemic)

There are 12 of these so-called cell salts. Based upon the ideas of a Dr Shuessler. They work on homoeopathic principles and are not true nutritional preparations. Available singly and in mixtures, they have no scientifically acceptable evidence to back their use. However, the wide consumer demand for products throughout the developed world must have more than folklore as its reason. Books on the system are available.

The tissue salts are:

> Calcium fluoride
> Calcium phosphate
> Calcium sulphate
> Iron phosphate
> Potassium chloride
> Potassium sulphate
> Potassium phosphate
> Magnesium phosphate
> Sodium chloride
> Sodium phosphate
> Sodium sulphate
> Silicic acid (silica)

■8 Amino acids

□*Introduction*

Amino acids are the basic molecular building blocks for proteins. Many millions of combinations are possible and because proteins play such a fundamental role in body processes, diets deficient in one or more of the essential amino acids can have adverse effects on health.

Many amino acids bind minerals closely to themselves and are known as chelating agents. Many products are available in health stores carrying the words 'chelated mineral' either as a major part of the title or as an aside. The superiority of these products over simple sulphates or chlorides is controversial. Since the proportion of minerals present is less as a percentage than in single salts, it is to be expected that they will be more digestible (see comments on page 116). Whether these minerals themselves reach their reactive sites in the body quicker or in a more appropriate form is unknown. Blood levels alone are not sufficient evidence for most scientists. It must be admitted that critics of the chelated minerals fail to produce criteria which they would accept. Too little is still known about mineral metabolism in the human body.

Specific effects of amino acid deficiency are difficult to assess and no official deficiency diseases exist apart from those associated with protein deficiency itself. Although amino acids are essential for life they are not documented like vitamins and minerals with RDAs and deficiency symptoms. Some nutritionists believe that altering amino acid dietary balance is wrong because the effects are not known. These people liken the amino acids to drugs. We believe that the body is well adapted to cope with widely varying amino acid combinations in the diet because of wide dietary differences. These differences must be experienced by individuals in their regular daily diets. So dietary regimes based upon increases in specific amino acids may help health conditions without the dangers associated with drugs.

Many drugs act by interfering with protein metabolism and possibly altering metabolic pathways normally lubricated by amino acids. Once altered those pathways may be permanently diverted to make either drug dependence or unpleasant side effects a reality. Even when available the natural amino acid or combination will not fit into the new pattern properly.

It seems that only limited research has been carried out on the benefits of amino acids in illnesses. This is probably because no patents can be obtained on their chemical structures. New drug substances are somewhat different commercially because they can be patented and give manufacturers monopoly powers. Even from the little evidence available it would appear that amino acids seem to have positive benefits without long term side effects. Tryptophan is a good example of an effective treatment which is safe but not successful as a drug since the commercial return is too small. Product competition was immediate upon the discovery of tryptophan's antidepressant effect. If a patent had been possible for the originator of the research, then he would have made a larger financial gain. Tryptophan's benefits were discovered around the same time that the benzodiazepine drugs were coming into vogue (valium, librium etc). Perhaps if tryptophan had been patentable then those drugs would not have succeeded. The patents provided the manufacturers with huge promotional budgets and enabled more similar drugs to be discovered. When there is only a little profit, knowledge progresses slowly, not kindled by the human drive for commercial success and power.

Supplementally, amino acid concentrates are generally taken apart from meals.

■Alanine

Non-essential. Body can make it for itself.α alanine.

□*Commercial sources for supplements*   All synthetically prepared by fairly simple chemical reactions.

□*Main functions*   Protein building. A potent stimulator of glucagon secretion from the pancreas and linked to glycogen release from the liver – hence the production of energy from body stores.

□*Deficiency symptoms*   None.

□*Co-factors*   None apart from other amino acids.

□*Overdosing and toxicity*   None.

□*RDA*   None, but if supplements are taken, not more than 2 g daily should be necessary.

Note: *Beta-alanine is used to synthesize pantothenic acid molecules but is not an amino acid used by the body.*

Alanine – good sources

* *best sources*
  * *maize flour (cornflour)
    lean beef
    tripe
    beefburgers
    meat paste
    fish
    crustacea
  * cauliflower
    spinach
  * meat extract spread
  * gelatin
    yeast extract
    yeast

■Arginine

Non-essential amino acid for adults, but may be essential for children.

□*Commercial sources* Synthetic chemical methods are used. The hydrochloride is commercially available as well as the free amino acid for supplement products.

□*Main functions* In detoxification processes for removing ammonia from the body through formation of urea in the liver. Stimulates the release of growth hormone from the pituitary, so is often recommended in body building programmes. Wound healing and collagen building needs arginine. It is anti-diuretic because it enables the body to make vasopressin, the anti-diuretic hormone secreted by the pituitary gland. Vasopressin is also said to be able to enhance memory. Arginine has a role in the immune system and may improve the body's resistance to infectious diseases. Like many other amino acids, arginine is involved in carbohydrate and fat metabolism as well as that of proteins.

□*Deficiency symptoms* None officially recognized, but many nutritionists believe that the modern diet is deficient in arginine and so term arginine as essential.

□*Co-factors* Ornithine, which is made by the body from arginine and can be converted back to it if necessary.

□*Overdosing and toxicity*   Arginine hydrochloride should not be administered to people suffering kidney or liver insufficiency problems. High doses of arginine may precipitate schizophrenic attacks and encourage the growth of herpes viruses.

□*RDA*   None. Doses of up to 4 g daily are used by some nutritionists but we would consider 2 g to be sufficient in any supplemental regime.

Arginine – good sources

best sources

    wheat bran
    rice
    soya flour
    egg yolk
    lean beef
    duck
    rabbit
    heart
    tripe
    corned beef
    ham
    tongue
    beefburgers
    prawn
    fish
    molluscs
  *broad beans
  *beetroot
  *cucumber
  *onions
  *peas
   chick peas
   spinach
  *grapes
   oranges
  *almonds
   brazils
   hazel nuts
   peanuts
   peanut butter
   plain chocolate
   gelatin

■Aspartic acid

Non-essential and not needed by the body for metabolism.

□*Commercial sources for supplements* Produced by the hydrolysis of synthetic asparagine, another non essential amino acid.

□*Main functions* Often used to carry minerals for supplementary purposes. Aspartates may be preferred dietary sources to simple inorganic sulphates or chlorides. This is probably because the concentration of the mineral within an aspartate salt is much less than in the inorganic salts (see page 116).

□*Deficiency symptoms* None.

□*Co-factors* None apart from other amino acids.

□*Overdosing and toxicity* None.

□*RDA* None. The amount of aspartic acid is usually determined by the amount of mineral aspartate used and it is the mineral part which will determine the dose used.

Aspartic acid – good sources

*best sources
      soya flour
      eggs
      lean beef
      fish
      crustacea
      molluscs
      asparagus
      French beans
      broad beans
      butter beans
      haricot beans
      red kidney beans
    *beetroot
      carrots
      lentils
      lettuce
      peas
      chick peas
      red pigeon peas
    *potatoes
      spinach

        tomatoes
      *apples
      *apricots
       bananas
      *figs
       grapes
       oranges
       pears
      *strawberries
       peanuts
       peanut butter
       plain chocolate
       yeast

(The very best source of aspartic acid from this list is beetroot with 1130 mg per g of nitrogen)

■Citrulline

Non-essential amino acid. Little documented and first isolated from water melon juice. Can be synthesized from arginine and ornithine.

■Cystine

Non-essential amino acid.

□*Commercial sources* Purified after hydrolysis of the hair protein keratin.

□*Main functions* Important in formation of the hair protein keratin and the blood sugar-controlling hormone insulin. May elevate cholesterol levels in blood. Sulphur-rich.

□*Deficiency symptoms* A genetically inherited metabolic disease, homocystinuria, is helped by a special diet rich in cystine and low in methionine.

□*Co-factors* None.

□*RDA* None. Cysteine supplements will provide cystine in the body (see page 146).

Cystine – good sources

best sources

　　　pearl barley
　　*wheat bran
　　　maize flour (cornflour)
　　*wheat flour
　　*oatmeal
　　*rice
　　　rye flour
　　　soya flour
　　　human milk
　　　eggs
　　　brain
　　　heart
　　　tripe
　　　molluscs
　　　spinach
　　*bananas
　　　dates
　　　figs
　　　grapes
　　　brazil nuts
　　　coconut
　　　walnuts
　　　plain chocolate
　　　cocoa
　　　beer

■Cysteine

Non-essential

□*Commercial sources*   From hydrolysis of proteins. Synthetic routes are also used but starting material is natural. The hydrochloride is the stable form.

□*Main functions*   A principal source of sulphur in the diet. Cysteine is used by the body to make taurine, the amino acid which combines with cholic acid to form a bile salt which aids fat digestion. May help iron absorption. Used in conjunction with calcium pantothenate to help some forms of arthritis. An integral part of the tripeptide glutathione (see page 176).

□*Deficiency symptoms*   None.

□*Co-factors*   Methionine, choline.

□*Overdosing and toxicity*   None.

□*RDA*   None. Supplements usually recommended allow for 200 to 1000 mg daily.

□*Stability*   In water free cysteine quickly breaks down to cystine (see page 144).

■Gamma amino butyric acid (GABA)

□*Commercial sources*   Synthesized by straightforward chemical methods.

□*Main functions*   Produced naturally in the body from glutamic acid and will have similar properties. Vitamin B6 is needed for its synthesis in the body. Has been used to lower blood pressure.

□*Overdosing and toxicity*   Large amounts can be taken with safety. 32 g is recorded as safe daily, although 8 g at once produced serious side effects of peripheral vascular collapse in one person.

□*RDA*   None. Normally supplements 250 to 500 mg and 2 or 3 tablets are used nutritionally.

■Glutamine and glutamic acid

L-glutamine is converted to L-glutamic acid in the body. L-glutamic acid hydrochloride may be considered similar nutritionally to L-glutamine.

□*Commercial forms for supplements*   Both L-glutamine and L-glutamic acid hydrochloride are produced synthetically for commercial use, but natural starting materials are often used.

□*Main functions*   L-glutamic acid hydrochloride, besides acting like L-glutamine, will also supply hydrochloric acid to the digestive system to aid protein digestion where acid deficiencies exist. Each 500 mg of L-glutamic acid hydrochloride yields 100 mg of hydrochloric acid. Glutamine is said to act as a brain fuel and is often recommended by nutritionists for patients with psychiatric problems and to help alcoholism. It may also help reduce craving for sugar. Glutamic acid is probably the active form in the brain, but glutamine is more efficiently transported in the body and therefore ultimately achieves high glutamic acid brain concentrations.

□*Deficiency symptoms* None officially recognized, but in the USA nutritionists believe that mental disorders and even drug dependence may be related to failure in glutamic acid biosynthesis in the body.

□*Co-factors* B group vitamins.

□*Overdosing and toxicity* None recorded. Maximum dosages mentioned as nutritional – 4 g daily. Normally some 1 to 2 g used.

□*Stability* Very stable.

Glutamic acid – good sources

*best sources
  pearl barley
  wheat bran
  *brown wheat flour
  *white wheat flour
  rye flour
  grapes
  almonds
  hazel nuts
  milk chocolate

■Glycine

Non-essential and the simplest of the amino acids.

□*Commercial sources* Synthesized by simple chemical reaction from acetic acid.

□*Main functions* Forms part of the haem pigment in red blood cells. Formation of bile salts and takes part in many detoxifying reactions within the body. It is used in the body processes which build the purine elements of nucleic acids.

□*Deficiency symptoms* None.

□*Co-factors* None.

□*Overdosing and toxicity* It is non-toxic and is often used as a base for chewable tablets to help make them 'melt' in the mouth.

□*RDA* None. Many grammes may be taken without any problem.

Glycine – good sources

*best sources

    wheat bran
    tripe
    tongue
    beefburgers
    brawn
    crustacea
    cauliflower
    *oranges
    hazel nuts
    *meat extract spread
    *gelatin

■Histidine

A non-essential amino acid, except for growing children.

□*Commercial sources for supplements* Chemically synthesized.

□*Main functions* A substance used by the body to produce histamine, which is released in allergic reactions and stimulates acid secretion in the stomach.

□*Deficiency symptoms* None.

□*Overdosing and toxicity*None.

□*RDA* None.

Histidine – good sources

*best sources

    lean bacon
    lean beef
    lean lamb
    lean pork
    brain
    kidney
    liver
    oxtail
    tongue
    ham

beefburgers
butterbeans
red pigeon peas
*bananas
grapes
milk chocolate
*gelatin

■Isoleucine

Essential, cannot be made by the body.

□*Commercial sources for supplements*   Isoleucine is made by purification and extraction processes from various sources, milk protein, egg protein, beet sugar and blood fibrin.

□*Main functions*   In the construction of body proteins generally.

□*Deficiency symptoms*   None apart from those associated with general protein deficiency.

□*Co-factors*   None apart from other amino acids.

□*Overdosing and toxicity*   None.

□*RDA*   None. Supplemental amounts up to 2 g daily should always be sufficient in supplemental regimes.

Isoleucine – good sources

*best sources

soya flour
*cow's milk
human milk
*yoghurt
*eggs
lean bacon
lean beef
lean pork
lean lamb
chicken
duck
turkey
rabbit
heart
tongue
corned beef

ham
veal
beefburgers
meat paste
crustacea
molluscs
butterbeans
spinach
*hazel nuts
*milk chocolate
yeast extracts
yeast

■Leucine

Essential amino acid.

□*Commercial sources*   Synthetic routes are used with final separation of the natural L form from the DL mixture.

□*Main functions*   The D form has been shown to have analgesic activity in animals. The natural L form is important in building enzymes and body proteins.

□*Deficiency symptoms*   None.

□*Co-factors*   None.

□*Overdosing and toxicity*   None.

□*RDA*   None. Supplements of 1 to 2 g are usually recommended.

Leucine – good sources

*best sources

Maize flour (cornflour)
oatmeal
rice
*cow's milk
human milk
yoghurt
eggs
lean beef
lean bacon
lean lamb
chicken
duck

turkey
rabbit
brain
heart
kidney
corned beef
ham
tongue
veal
beefburgers
meat paste
fish
crustacea
molluscs
butterbeans
haricot beans
red kidney beans
lentils
chick peas
*spinach
*walnuts
*milk chocolate
yeast

■Lysine

Essential amino acid found mainly in animal proteins.

□*Commercial sources* All synthetically produced. Can be isolated by acid hydrolysis of proteins but this is not economic compared with chemical synthesis. Usual form is lysine hydrochloride.

□*Main functions* Growth, tissue repair, production of many body proteins. Has been recommended as a preventative and controller of herpes infection, but evidence is conflicting and the treatment is not accepted by most doctors. Holistic practitioners will include supplements in their overall treatment regimes. Considerable excess of lysine over arginine may be important in this respect (see Arginine, page 141). Migraines and even Bell's palsy have been helped with lysine. It can be converted to carnitine in the body and has reduced blood cholesterol levels in animal experiments.

□*Deficiency symptoms* Tiredness, poor concentration, irritability, bloodshot eyes, hair loss – general health problems associated with protein deficiency. Lysine is lacking in cereal proteins, thus people depending on these items for their protein intake may require extra lysine in their diet as a supplement (vegans in particular).

□*Co-factors*   None, apart from other amino acids.

□*Overdosing and toxicity*   Large doses of lysine hydrochloride, over 2 g at once, will cause acidosis.

□*RDA*   None. Supplements containing 500 mg are usually used and two or three tablets a day are generally a sufficient supplementary allowance.

Lysine – good sources

*best sources
>   lean beef
> *lean lamb
> *lean pork
>   chicken
>   duck
>   turkey
>   rabbit
>   brain
>   oxtail
>   tongue
>   corned beef
> *fish

■Methionine

Essential amino acid. Has a characteristic pungent and unpleasant odour and is a sulphur-containing amino acid.

□*Commercial sources for supplements*   All synthesized chemically. Usual form is DL methionine but L-methionine is the natural form.

□*Main functions*   A chelator of the toxic heavy metals, and helps remove them from the body. Speeds formation of the tripeptide glutathione (see page 176). Used as an antidote in paracetamol poisoning. (Paracetamol is a drug widely used as a pain killer and is available both on prescription and over the counter in chemist shops. It can also be found in low doses in some products available in health stores.) Used to lower urinary pH (make it more acid). It is helpful in the breaking down of fats (a lipotropic agent). It is important in the formation of the blood proteins called globulins and albumins. It is also said to reduce cholesterol deposits in arteries.

□*Deficiency symptoms*   Fatty liver, but on its own seldom corrects this, and other factors are required, for example choline. Hair loss.

□*Co-factors*   Choline, folic acid.

□*Overdosing and toxicity*   Should not be given as an antidote to paracetamol more than 10 hours after the overdose. Doses of over 5 g may cause nausea and vomiting in some people.

□*RDA*   None. Supplemental regimes 500 to 1000 mg are usually recommended daily.

Methionine – good sources

*best sources
    *cow's milk
     eggs
     lean bacon
    *lean beef
     lean lamb
    *lean pork
     chicken
    *duck
    *turkey
     rabbit
     liver
     tripe
     corned beef
     tongue
    *ham
     veal
    *beefburgers
     meat paste
    *fish
     crustacea
     molluscs
    *grapes
    *peaches
     brazil nuts

(Grapes and peaches on this list should be of interest to vegetarians and vegans.)

■Ornithine

□*Natural sources*   A free amino acid found in body tissues, but not used as a building block for proteins.

□*Commercial sources for supplements*   Prepared and purified from natural sources.

□*Main functions*   A hormone releaser. It influences fat burning and muscle growth through release of growth hormone and insulin. It is also said to influence the immune system and may help reduce arterial fatty plaque deposits. It has been used in diets for sufferers from atherosclerosis/heart disease.

□*Deficiency systems*   To occur, the body will lack arginine in the diet because it makes ornithine from that amino acid. In diets deficient in protein, ornithine levels will be affected so will all the other amino acid-dependent body proteins.

□*Co-factors*   Arginine, from which it is made. Glutamic acid and proline which can be made from it.

□*Overdosing and toxicity*   None in the amounts used nutritionally of 250 mg to 2 g daily.

□*RDA*   Not an officially recognized nutrient, but supplementally 500 to 1000 mg daily should prove adequate within an overall dietary control regime.

□*Stability*   Ornithine is stable in supplements.

■L-Phenylalanine

Essential amino acid.

□*Commercial sources for supplements*   Prepared by separation after hydrolysis of proteins such as lactalbumin and zein (corn protein).

□*Main functions*   Converted to tyrosine in the body so has similar actions (see page 161). Said to help mental processes and depress appetite. The D form has been found to have pain-killing effects (see DL Phenylalanine, page 155).

□*Deficiency symptoms*   None. If the enzyme which converts phenylalanine to tyrosine is absent, then health problems develop. The disease is known as phenylketonuria. If children with this disease are not fed diets low in phenylalanine, then serious mental retardation occurs. Special diet foods are available to treat this disease.

□*Co-factors*   None.

□*Overdosing and toxicity*   None, apart from phenylketonuria as above.

□*RDA*   None. 500 to 2000 mg are usually recommended as suitable supplemental intakes.

L-Phenylalanine–good sources

*best sources

> pearl barley
> maize flour (cornflour)
> white wheat flour
> oatmeal
> rice
> soya flour
> cow's milk
> yoghurt
> eggs
> *egg white
> brain
> kidney
> oxtail
> tongue
> *butterbeans
> haricot beans
> lentils
> lettuce
> *chickpeas
> *red pigeon peas
> *spinach
> peanuts
> *milk chocolate

■DL-Phenylalanine

Also known as DLPA, but this is not an official generic abbreviation.

□*Commercial sources*   Prepared by synthetic processes.

□*Main functions*   D-phenylalanine is a pain killer which is said to work by stimulation of the body's own pain-killing endorphins. It does not work immediately but over a period which may be up to a month. The mixture DLPA is weaker than the D form but much more economic and also provides the essential L-phenylalanine to help general body metabolism (see page 154). It may be taken in conjunction with pain killers like aspirin and paracetamol which give a quicker effect and these may be stopped when DLPA has completed its job.

□*Co-factors*   D-leucine.

□*Overdosing and toxicity*   Precautions will apply as for phenylalanine (see page 154).

□*RDA*   None. Supplements with strengths of 375 mg appear to be the norm. 2 of these 3 times daily are usually recommended.

□*Bibliography DLPA to end Chronic Pain and Depression* (Longshadow Books, New York).

■Proline

Non-essential, may be synthesized within the body

□*Commercial sources for supplements*   Several synthetic methods are available. No commercial proline is extracted from proteins.

□*Main functions*   Associated with the condition of connective tissue – collagen building. It is important in skin health and posture. Injury to soft tissue may be helped by a high proline diet.

□*Deficiency symptoms*   None officially accepted

□*Co-factors*   Vitamin C and other amino acids.

□*Overdosing and toxicity*   None.

□*RDA*   None, but a supplementary regime with up to 2 g daily should be sufficient.

Proline – good sources

*best sources
      pearl barley
      maize flour (cornflour)
      wholewheat flour
      brown flour
     *white flour
      rye flour
      cow's milk

          human milk
          tripe
          milk chocolate
        *beer
        *lager
          meat extract spread
        *gelatin

■Serine

Non-essential.

□*Commercial sources* Synthetic routes available but demand for pure serine for commercial purpose is low. Its role in the body metabolism is not documented. No deficiency symptoms or co-factors. Nutritional supplements of 500 mg are available.

Serine – good sources

best sources
          wheat bran
          maize flour (cornflour)
          wheat flours
          soya flour
          cow's milk
          yoghurt
        *eggs
          brain
          heart
          kidney
          fish
          molluscs
          crustacea
          French beans
        *butter beans
          haricot beans
          red kidney beans
          lentils
          chick peas
          spinach
          grapes
        *hazel nuts
          coconut
          peanuts

peanut butter
milk chocolate
plain chocolate
yeast extract
yeast

■Taurine

Non-essential and not found in dietary proteins. Made from cysteine by the body.

□*Natural sources* Marine animals, especially molluscs – mussels, oysters, snails and octopus. Organ meats, especially brain.

□*Commercial sources for supplements* Synthetically produced by straightforward chemical methods.

□*Main functions* Forms a bile acid with glycocholic acid to help digestion of fats. Works against fatty degeneration of the liver. Its role in heart problems and nervous problems such as epilepsy is controversial. Essential for normal development of babies. It is found in high concentrations in brain tissue and is said to assist in helping alcoholics wishing to overcome their addiction.

□*Deficiency* Will occur if metabolic disturbance does not allow cysteine to be converted to taurine efficiently.

□*Co-factors* Choline, vitamins B1 and B2. Methionine in detoxification processes.

□*Overdosing and toxicity* None. Doses of 7 g daily have been given to help epilepsy. 6 g daily for congestive heart failure (*Current Therapeutic Research*, 34, 543, 1983).

□*RDA* None.

■Threonine

Essential amino acid.

□*Commercial sources* Pure L-threonine can be produced synthetically and by separation after protein hydrolysis.

□*Main functions* As an essential part of many body proteins and enzymes.

□*Deficiency symptoms* None.

158

□*Co-factors* None.

□*Overdosing and toxicity* None.

□*RDA* None. Supplemental regimes including 500 to 2000 mg daily are used by some nutritionists.

Threonine – good sources

*best sources

> human milk
> yoghurt
> *eggs
> lean bacon
> lean beef
> lean lamb
> lean pork
> chicken
> duck
> turkey
> rabbit
> *brain
> heart
> kidney
> oxtail
> tongue
> tripe
> corned beef
> ham
> veal
> meat paste
> beefburgers
> *fish
> *crustacea
> *molluscs
> butterbeans

■Tryptophan

Essential.

□*Commercial sources* Synthetic methods are used.

□*Main functions* As a starting material for the body to build its own vitamin B3 (nicotinamide). Precursor of important neurotransmitter 5HT (5-hydroxy-tryptamine) also known as serotonin. Depressive conditions appear to be related to serotonin concentrations in the brain and tryptophan has been used to help these conditions. Also aids sleep. Tryptophan has been found to lower cholesterol levels in blood in animals. Migraine and pain relief have also been helped.

□*Deficiency symptoms*   None, but see Vitamin B3, page 75.

□*Co-factors*   Vitamin B6 and vitamin C.

□*Overdosing and toxicity*   Since tryptophan has effects on the nervous system, overdosing may cause problems. Drowsiness, nausea and anorexia have been reported. However, these are quickly reversed by reduction in dosage and none of the addictive problems associated with tranquillizers and sleeping drugs arises. The body knows how to cope with tryptophan and no metabolic pathways are diverted by its use. Meals high in tryptophan have similar effects. High carbohydrate meals in combination with low protein stimulate serotonin production. However, if high protein meals with extra tryptophan are taken, less serotonin is produced because of competition with other amino acids. So for maximum effect with tryptophan, use a moderate high carbohydrate, low protein diet. (A booklet on suitable diets to combine with Tryptophan has been written.[1])

□*Warning*   Monoamine Oxidase inhibitor drugs are incompatible with tryptophan and they should not be taken together. The drugs are phenelzine (nardil), parnate, parstelin, eutonyl. Tryptophan should not be taken during pregnancy.

□*RDA*   None. 500 mg three times a day with a suitable diet for use as an anti-depressant. 1 to 2 g half an hour before retiring for sleep. 5 g may be taken as a single dose, but beware of drowsiness.

Tryptophan – good sources

*best sources

> pearl barley
> cow's milk
> human milk
> eggs
> corned beef
> French beans
> potatoes
> spinach

[1]   *Anxiety, Depression and Nutrition*, Dr Barrie Bartlett (Roberts Publications, London, 1983).

*dates
hazel nuts
dates
peanut butter
*milk chocolate
plain chocolate
*beer
*lager

(Lager is an exceptionally high source of tryptophan at 410 mg per g of nitrogen)

∎L-Tyrosine

Non-essential. Formed in the body from phenylalanine.

□*Commercial sources for supplements* By separation after hydrolysis of casein or zein (corn protein).

□*Main functions* Essential in formation of adrenaline, thyroxine and the hair pigment melanin. Whilst the body can make it from phenylalanine, some 70% of daily need is directly available from protein digestion. It is said to help depression associated with taking the contraceptive pill. The neurotransmitters produced from it are often in deficiency in Parkinson-type illnesses. It is claimed to depress appetite and so may help slimmers. Anxiety and depression which are drug resistant have been helped. May lower raised blood pressure but equally it can be used to raise blood pressure to normal if it has been depressed by shock caused by severe loss of blood.

□*Deficiency symptoms* None officially recognized, but tyrosine's wide use in body protein building makes it a very important element despite being termed 'non-essential'.

□*Overdosing and toxicity* None.

□*Co-factors* Phenylalanine and tryptophan.

□*RDA* None. Nutritional doses of 2 to 3 g daily are not uncommon in supplemental regimes.

Tyrosine – good sources
*best sources
    maize flour (cornflour)
    oatmeal

    *rice
    cow's milk
    yoghurt
    eggs
    lean bacon
    lean beef
    lean lamb
    lean pork
    chicken
    duck
    turkey
    rabbit
    brain
    oxtail
    corned beef
    ham
    tongue
    veal
    beefburgers
    fish
    *crustacea
    *molluscs
    French beans
    broad beans
    butter beans
    broccoli tops
    lentils
    onions
    *spinach
    figs
    pears
    strawberries
    hazel nuts
    peanuts
    walnuts
    milk chocolate
    yeast

■Valine

Essential amino acid.

□*Commercial sources*   Chemically synthesized.

□*Main functions*   Constituent of proteins, particularly fibrous ones.

□*Deficiency symptoms*   None.

□*Co-factors*   None.

□*Overdosing and toxicity*   None.

□*RDA*   None. Supplements in tablet form of 500 mg are available.

Valine – good sources

best sources
      rice
      *cow's milk
      yoghurt
      *eggs
      brain
      heart
      kidney
      liver
      fish
      molluscs
      milk chocolate
      yeast extract
      *yeast

■9 Enzymes and miscellaneous factors

■Enzymes

Scientific progress has led to the isolation and commercial availability of several enzymes. All are proteins and largely destroyed by digestive processes. In order to ensure an enzyme enters the bloodstream, it must be injected. However, this does not ensure its activity, because the true site of action is often a considerable distance from the injected point and the enzyme could be destroyed on the way there. Some enzymes are only produced momentarily at their reactive site, e.g. inside particular organ cells, such as the liver and kidney. Enzymes which act in the digestive tract may be considered as nutrients in the broadest sense. We have included some comments on a few of the better-known ones. Attempts to ensure enzyme products reach their appropriate sites of action in the digestive system are usually made. This is done by special attention to capsule and tablet protective coatings.

Pepsin

The stomach enzyme often taken with betaine hydrochloride. It is a protein digester prepared from ox or pig stomach juices.

Lactase

The milk digestive enzyme prepared by extraction processes from animal tissues. Used to help people who cannot tolerate lactose (milk sugar). Lactose is found in milk and is also added as a filler to capsules and tablets, which makes the declaration of all ingredients in drugs and supplements very important to help lactose-sensitive people.

164

Amylase

A group of starch-digesting enzymes usually isolated commercially from pancreas glands. There are several types. Alpha-amylase is one, and when there was a vogue for starch-blocker slimming products some years ago, it was an alpha-amylase inhibitor which was promoted for the purpose. Its effectiveness was never proved.

Lipase

A group of fat-digesting enzymes usually isolated from pancreas glands. It is activated by vitamin C, glutathione and cysteine.

Rennin

The milk-clotting enzyme found in babies' stomachs. After weaning, production of the enzyme ceases. Rennet is the commercial powder containing rennin and is prepared from calf stomachs or by fermentation using certain non-pathogenic bacteria. Rennet tablets are sold to make junket custards and cheeses.

■Super oxide dismutases (SOD)

□*Natural sources* Enzymes which are found throughout the body. Sources include seafood, meat, poultry and organ meats.

□*Commercial sources for supplements* Derived from bovine (bull) tissues and purified and separated by special enzymatic concentrating processes. The potency of the final product, which always contains catalase too, is expressed in MFU, which are units of activity.

□*Main functions* As free radical neutralizers. Protect cells and said to be anti-aging enzymes. SOD levels in the body are said to reduce with age, and this in turn increases the signs of aging caused by unchecked free radical activity – wrinkles, supple connective tissues turning fibrous, joint problems.

□*Deficiency symptoms* Signs of aging.

□*Co-factors* Vitamin E, selenium, copper, zinc, manganese.

□*Overdosing and toxicity* By mouth most scientists believe enzymes to be ineffective because they are broken down by the digestive enzymes of the stomach. SOD enzymes also work within cells and cannot cross cell membranes. However, some free radicals will be found ouside cells and even in the digestive tract, so oral SOD may help the body cope at these sites, leaving its natural resources to concentrate on SOD production within cells. SOD is non-toxic. It is also used by injection. Even by this route it cannot get into cells but may assist the body by working in the extra-cellular tissue against free radicals. SOD enzymes provide the organic forms of minerals such as copper, zinc and manganese and it may be that these contribute to its beneficial effects when taken as tablets or capsules.

□*RDA* None. Supplements are now available yielding 5000 units of activity per dose. A dose regime of 2000 to 10,000 units daily is usually recommended.

□*Stability* In supplements SOD is fairly stable at normal temperature but will be destroyed by excessive heat.

■Bromelain

□*Natural source* Pineapples.

□*Commercial forms for supplement* Bromelain is prepared by concentration and extraction from pineapple juice. It is standardized by reference to GDU (units of enzyme activity in the digestion of protein).

□*Main functions* As a meat tenderizer and an aid to protein digestion in the acid conditions of the stomach.

□*Deficiency symptoms* None.

□*Co-factors* Often used in conjunction with papain, the enzyme from the paw-paw plant (papaya).

□*Overdosing and toxicity* Usually contained in minute amounts in protein mixtures for diet supplement purposes. Concentrated supplements containing the enzyme in tablet or capsule form should be taken after or with food. Normal dosage of 100 to 200 mg. Large amounts may cause nausea and sickness. There have been a few reports of allergic reactions to this natural extract.

□*Stability* Very stable.

■Papaya

The dried paw-paw fruit is rich in the enzyme papain. This enzyme is a protein digester and is used to tenderize meat.

□*Main functions* To help digestion. Naturopaths prefer this and the pineapple enzyme, bromelain, to treat patients with digestive problems. Orthodox doctors would treat these same people with chemical antacids.

□*Supplemental form* Usually in chewable fruit flavoured tablets but may be swallowed as a simple tablet after meals as a digestive aid.

■Acidophilus

□*Natural and commercial sources* Yoghurt bacteria, milk-grown lactobacillus acidophilus. Some non-milk grown bacilli are also available but are much more expensive and are designed to help those people who cannot tolerate milk-based foods.

□*Main functions* The acidophilus family of bacteria are friendly to the human system. They live in the large intestine, helping destroy toxins and producing vitamins as by-products. They have been used within holistic treatment regimes to help 'thrushes' (a form of fungal infection) and allergies.

□*Deficiency symptoms* Foul stools, excessive flatulence, bad breath, poor digestion. After a course of antibiotics or sulpha drugs, which are used medically to kill pathogenic organisms (the unfriendly invaders responsible for infectious diseases), the friendly acidophilus are killed also. Taking yoghurt and acidophilus-based supplements makes sense after completion of the drug course to re-establish the friendly bacterial population quickly.

□*Co-factors* Fibre, lactose, pectin.

□*Overdosing and toxicity* None.

□*RDA* Supplements usually contain at least 1,000,000 viable organisms, but preferably 10,000,000. Powders are generally more potent because the tabletting process kills organisms, but tablets are more convenient to use for many people.

□*Stability* Acidophilus supplements should be stored in a refrigerator at below 4°C. Shelf life of tablets is about twelve months in such conditions.

■Aloe vera

This is an extract from the leaves of a lily family cactus.

□*Main functions*   Used in cosmetics to assist healing of burns and injuries, also to improve skin and hair condition. Internally, it has been used as a food supplement with claimed but unproven beneficial effects on digestion and relief of gastric ulcers. It contains vitamin C and minerals, topped with many micronutrients.

□*Deficiency symptoms*   None.

□*Co-factors*   Polyunsaturated fatty acids, vitamin E.

□*Overdosing and toxicity*   None.

□*RDA*   None. There are no standardization procedures regarding its manufacture, so wide variations in properties are to be expected.

■Alfalfa

□*Natural source*   Lucerne, a leguminous plant, growing with very deep roots. Alfalfa seeds are often used as sprouters for macrobiotic diets.

□*Commercial forms*   The Lucerne (stem and leaves only) is dried before incorporation into tablets or capsules.

□*Main functions*   As a rich source of minerals and vitamins. It is rich in vitamins K, A, B6 and E. It is used by herbalists for both its laxative and diuretic properties.

□*Deficiency symptoms*   As a rich source of vitamins and minerals it is often used as a basic supplement to correct minor deficiencies.

□*Overdosing and toxicity*   None, but large amounts of dried herb may lead to very loose stools.

□*Stability*   Very stable as dried herb.

■Bee products

The honey bee has been exploited by man through the centuries for its honey. This natural sweet substance has had magical life-enhancing properties ascribed to it. More recently, other bee products have been introduced to us by the health food industry, including royal jelly, bee collected pollen and propolis. All these products are claimed to have health-giving properties, but there is little scientifically acceptable evidence to back them. This does not mean that they are not beneficial as their proponents claim. Proof is elusive and is likely to continue to be so.

☐*Honey*

A food produced from plant nectar to enable the general hive population to thrive. It is a water-based syrup of glucose and fructose with trace factors including vitamins, minerals and enzymes. It has been used as a basis of many home remedies for coughs and colds. It has therefore passed into medicinal folklore.

There is no scientific evidence to support its use or benefits. Any research programme would be extremely costly. Honeys come from all over the world where different plant populations exist, so finding a reference base could prove a big stumbling block for any research. It is high in glucose content and therefore potentially harmful to teeth.

☐*Pollen*

Pollens are the sperms of the flowering plant world. Bees collect pollens as well as nectar from plants. They feed their larvae on pollen and a very rapid growth rate of some 1500 times in six days takes place.

Pollens contain the eight essential amino acids as well as a host of vitamins, minerals and micronutrient co-factors.

The longevity and health of people who live in the Azerbajan region of Russia has been attributed to their regular ingestion of pollen-rich honey scrap from their bee hives. Pollen is also claimed to help prostatis (inflammation of the prostate gland) and assist in athletic performance.

There is a great amount of anecdotal evidence of the benefits of pollens in the diet, but because the material itself is so variable there is no valid scientific research behind it. It is unlikely that scientific proof as to its benefits will ever exist. However, pollens are safe to use provided you are not allergic to them. Hayfever and asthma sufferers should be particularly wary of pollen supplements. May well prove a useful dietary addition to improve general health and wellbeing.

☐*Propolis*

This is a bee-produced substance which seals the part of the hive where the young are to be reared, and protects the larvae from infection. Claims have been made that propolis is a powerful infection fighter not only for bee progeny but also for humans. It is marketed in lozenges as a treatment for mouth and throat infections. It is also put into creams to assist healing burns, sprains and bruises. Valid scientific evidence for the effectiveness of propolis is not available. Much anecdotal detail exists, with many devotees. Could belief in the magic power of the bee be responsible?

□*Royal Jelly*

The most expensive bee product. The food of the queen bee, the most important member of the highly organized hive. Produced by worker bees, this substance makes her fertile and ensures a long and healthy life. Will it do this for you? Unlikely. No scientific evidence suggests that anything but a complex mixture of ingredients exists.

Royal Jelly has been discounted as a worthwhile nutrient but sales in the developed world produce good revenues for China. Some scientific work in the early 1960s suggested that in a mixture with pantothenic acid it could help arthritis sufferers. Costs, ridicule and shortage of reliable material meant that this work was never followed up.

■Betaine

□*Natural sources* Beet molasses.

□*Commercial form used in supplements* Betaine hydrochloride produced synthetically.

□*Main functions* In the hydrochloride form it provides hydrochloric acid to the extent of approximately 25% of its weight. It is used in supplements to increase the acid content of the stomach and to aid protein digestion. It aids vitamin C absorption and protects B vitamins.

□*Deficiency symptoms* If hydrochloric acid is secreted in lesser amounts than digestive processes need, then nutritional yields from foods may be depressed.

□*Co-factors* Stomach enzymes, vitamin C.

□*Overdosing and toxicity* Since betaine hydrochloride yields hydrochloric acid in the stomach, it should be used cautiously. Always after meals on a full stomach and preferably dissolved in water. This avoids local over-concentration and subsequent irritation to the stomach. Maximum amount to be taken at one time should not exceed 1.2 g. It should not be used by peptic ulcer sufferers.

□*RDA* There is none. However, it is said that as we grow older, less hydrochloric acid is secreted naturally and therefore many people over 40 would be helped by adding a supplement containing betaine hydrochloride to their diet.

□*Stability* Very stable as the hydrochloride. Betaine itself quickly absorbs water from the air to form a saturated solution.

■Bicarbonates

□*Commercial sources* Sodium and potassium bicarbonate powders.

□*Main functions* As rapid neutralizers of over-acidity in the body. People suffering severe allergy to foodstuffs may be helped by quickly taking about 2 g of bicarbonates of soda or potassium.

□*Deficiency symptoms* Not applicable.

□*Overdosing and toxicity* The body can correct itself after large intakes of bicarbonate but it is not advisable to take more than 5 g at any one time.

□*RDA* None.

■Charcoal

□*Natural sources* Burning of sawdust and other vegetable matter in such a way as to make a fine powder with a large adsorptive capacity. Charcoal can be prepared from animal bones but animal charcoal is not as efficient as a cleanser as the vegetable-derived kind.

□*Main functions* As an adsorbent of toxic waste materials in the intestines. It is not absorbed as a nutrient.

□*Deficiency symptoms* None.

□*Co-factors* Acidophilus – whilst the charcoal cleanses poisons from the gut, the acidophilus re-seeds the friendly bacteria once more.

□*Overdosing and toxicity* Purity standards for charcoal are important. Edible and medicinal varieties must meet strict requirements as regards content of toxic minerals. The letters BP or USP after the charcoal denote such quality.

□*Stability* Very stable.

■Chlorophyll

Chlorophyll is a mixture of complex highly coloured substances.

□*Natural sources*   All green plants. Chlorophyll is mainly concentrated in the leaves.

□*Commercial forms for supplements*   All commercial chlorophylls are prepared by extraction from dried green plants.

□*Main functions*   As a natural colour in cosmetics and foods. It contains chelated magnesium and is a natural source of that mineral. Has been used as a breath deodorant, although there is no satisfactory proof of its effectiveness.

□*Deficiency symptoms*   When plant leaves go yellow, the chlorophyll has been lost.

□*Co-factors*   It has been described as the 'haemoglobin' of the plant world.

□*Overdosing and toxicity*   None.

□*Stability*   Dried chlorophyll is very stable.

■Chondroitin sulphate A (CSA)

Long-chain mucropolysaccharides.

□*Natural sources*   Animal connective tissue.

□*Commercial sources*   Purified extracted cartilage. The factor chondroitin sulphate B is found in skin, arterial walls and heart tissue.

□*Main functions*   To provide essential bonding between the protein filaments. Pure extracted CSA has been used to treat heart disease and osteo-arthritis.

□*Deficiency symptoms*   None recognized.

□*Co-factors*   None.

□*Overdosing and toxicity*   None.

□*RDA*   None. CSA is likely to be substantially digested in the body to its component parts. Evidence of effects are lacking at present but the compounds may in future prove as interesting as lecithins.

■Devil's claw

A herbal preparation from the root of the South African plant Harpagophytum procumbens. Many herbalists believe it to have anti-arthritic properties, but the active ingredient remains unknown. It is frequently used within an overall holistic programme of diet for treatment of rheumatic conditions. As a root it is naturally rich in minerals and fibre.

■Dolomite

A natural source of calcium and magnesium in the form of calcium magnesium carbonate (500 mg of dolomite yields approximately 108 mg calcium and 66 mg magnesium). The food supplement quality material should be virtually free from heavy metals, such as lead and contaminants such as arsenic. It is sometimes used in supplements as a source of minerals and a neutralizer of the acidity associated with vitamin C.

■DMSO/dimethyl sulphoxide

□*Natural sources* None.

□*Synthetic and commercial forms* Chemically prepared from by-products of wood pulp.

□*Main functions* DMSO is a controversial substance with many properties claimed but with no substantiation. It is not a nutrient and no health store should offer it. The authors have found it in US stores on vitamin shelves but labelled DMSO solvent.

□*Deficiency* Impossible.

□*Co-factors* It has been used as a potentiator of drug action because it can make some cell membranes more permeable to some drug substances.

□*Overdosing and toxicity* It is a skin irritant. Blindness has been produced in animal experiments using it. Its use in cosmetics is prohibited in Britain.

□*Stability* Very stable, but hygroscopic (picks up water).

■Gelatin

A protein derived from animal bones. Used to prepare the shells of soft and hard capsules in conjunction with additives like glycerin. Many commercial grades are available, and the actual grade used is often vital to the success of subsequent food processing.

As a protein food, gelatin is not of good nutritional status as it does not contain the amino acids lysine or tryptophan. Gelatin has been recommended as a specific food supplement for preventing and curing brittle finger nails. The basis of this claim is not considered scientifically acceptable, but as a base for a general 'healthy nail' formula combining other vitamins (A and D) and minerals (calcium and zinc), there is probably positive benefit.

Gelatin as a food is completely safe, but like gelatin capsules, is unsuitable for vegetarians and vegans.

■Garlic

□*Natural sources*   Garlic bulb – Allium sativum (Liliaceae).

□*Commercial forms*   Garlic oil contains a large number of components including essential fatty acids, some B vitamins and vitamin C. The odour comes from allicin derivatives. Odourless garlic is now available where the fresh bulbs have been processed to prevent the development of the odour-producing compounds. Claims of the superiority of odourless forms over the normal oil are not widely accepted but much research continues into this most interesting of the 'health giving' herbs.

□*Main functions*   As an internal purifier (Russian penicillin) and protector against heart and circulatory disorders. It is claimed to help lower both blood pressure and cholesterol levels. Many herbalists use it routinely in treating colds, sore throats and running noses. It has been found to lower blood glucose and may help diabetics.

□*Deficiency symptoms*   Not relevant, but it would probably be a good idea for everyone to eat a meal liberally seasoned with garlic every day.

□*Co-factors*   Parsley is often used to counteract the odour of garlic in cooking and tablets.

□*Overdosing and toxicity*   None recorded, but direct contact of garlic oil with skin may produce allergic reaction in some people.

□*Stability*   In air, fresh cut garlic soon develops a strong odour, but there is no evidence that its nutritional value is diminished.

■Ginsengs

There are many types of ginseng, including Korean Red, Chinese White, Siberian, American, Indian; and Dong Quai is also grouped with the ginsengs.

□*Commercial forms*   Whole, cut or powdered roots. Some standardized extracts are commercially available but the basis of their standardization does not satisfy many scientists.

□*Main functions*   Ginsengs are used by herbalists and nutritionists as adaptogens. These are substances which are claimed to help the body correct itself. Ginsengs may be used medicinally for helping patients with apparently opposite symptoms. Some herbalists recommend the root of Dong Quai as an adaptogen for women in preference to ginseng. The active constituents of ginseng are said to be a group of saponins known as ginsenosides.

□*Deficiency symptoms*   Not applicable.

□*Co-factors*   Ginsengs are used in many proprietary tonics in combination with vitamin E and minerals. Several of the brands have been very successful and have established international consumer acceptance.

□*Overdosing and toxicity*   Side effects with ginseng have been widely reported, even dependence in a few people. Long-term ingestion of doses exceeding 2 g of dried root daily should be avoided.

Some standardized preparations based upon extracts of ginseng roots are available, and this makes dosing, at least, more reproducible. So much adulteration of ginseng has taken place that the Korean government has instituted control in many ways similar to the 'appellation controlée' associated with French wines. Even so, widespread variation in quality is a major obstacle to acceptance of ginseng as a valuable addition to medicine's or nutrition's armamentarium.

□*Stability*   Whole roots maintain their properties for a long time, but it is said that the powdering operation considerably reduces ginseng's potency.

■Glandulars and specific animal organs

Many organs can be separated from slaughtered animals. Over time, special medical uses have been found for many of these organs. The glands have proved rich sources of hormones and folklore. Bull's prostate and testes were obvious candidates for sexual potency enhancers, whilst ovary was a female health problem solver. The fact that after slaughter and processing hormones in many dried glands were undetectable did not prevent their use and recommendation for medicinal purposes.

Scientific progress enabled the isolation of the hormones and the production of synthetic substitutes. Many of these have yielded real progress. The corticosteroids from suprarenal glands is one, and thyroxine from thyroid is another; the sex hormone oestradiol developed from ovarian hormone, whilst the male sex hormone testosterone came from development of the active hormone in the testes. As a result of this progress many dried whole glandular extracts are closely controlled as medicinal substances and cannot be used as specific nutrients. Their very low activity, when compared with corresponding pure synthetic hormones, is ignored.

In the USA many nutritionally oriented practitioners are using dried glands and organs in their dietary therapies. They contend that use of a carefully prepared organ extract will assist the corresponding organ of the body to regenerate itself. This is achieved, they believe, by the whole nutrient spectrum being provided. The presence of hormones in the extract is not important. It is the other factors unrecognized by scientists that they believe are really vital. They claim that they stimulate the patient's corresponding organ into working more efficiently. Such practitioners give brain powder for memory, pancreas for diabetes, heart for blood and circulatory problems, spinal cord for nerve problems etc., etc. It must be emphasized that these items are not given in isolation but as part of a whole nutritional approach.

■Glutathione

A tripeptide consisting of glutamic acid, cysteine and glycine.

□*Commercial form* It can be isolated from yeast but is normally synthesized using fairly complex methods.

□*Main functions* The active part of the molecule is the SH group from cysteine. It is a detoxifier, antioxidant and deactivator of free radicals. Prolongs cell life and is included in most of the life extension dietary programmes recommended in the USA. Claims which are not well substantiated include anti-cancer, protection against the effects of tobacco smoke, radiation and X-rays. Said to help in the utilization of iron to a greater extent than vitamin C.

□*Deficiency symptoms* None recognized. Proponents claim that as we grow older, less glutathione is produced naturally in the body and therefore they say we need to take extra.

□*Co-factors*   Vitamin E, vitamin C.

□*Overdosing and toxicity*   None.

□*RDA*   None. Nutritionists recommend supplements yielding 150 to 300 mg daily. Reports indicate that glutathione is absorbed if taken by mouth (A.M. Novi, R. Florke, and N. Stukenkempfer, N.Y. Acad. Sci., 1982).

■Haemoglobin

The natural red pigment of red blood cells.

□*Natural source*   Dry blood.

□*Commercial forms*   Haemoglobin is prepared by a special extraction and drying process from whole blood – usually ox blood.

□*Main functions*   As a source of natural chelated iron. It is the best nutritional source of iron from the animal kingdom.

□*Deficiency symptoms*   Anaemia, pale skin and fatigue (see Iron, page 116).

□*Co-factors*   Folic acid, vitamin B12 and vitamin C.

□*Overdosing and toxicity*   None.

□*Stability*   Dried haemoglobin is very stable.

■Kelp

A general term for seaweed supplements, although there was a standard kelp called Kelpware BPC, made from Fucus vesiculosus, officially recognized some years ago.

□*Commercial sources for supplements*   Various species of Fucus – bladderwrack seaweeds. Those from deep unpolluted oceans are preferred. Irish Sea, Baltic Sea and Pacific Ocean are just a few of the more popular areas for harvesting nutritional seaweeds.

□*Main functions*   As a dietary source of most trace minerals, particularly iodine.

□*Deficiency symptoms*   See Iodine (page 115).

□*Overdosing and toxicity*   Some varieties of kelp are adjusted for iodine content using mineral iodides. Too much free iodine is undesirable.

□*RDA* Depends upon iodine content which is normally about 200 mcg organic iodine per 300 mg tablet. Up to 6 tablets normally used supplementally.

■Lecithin

Lecithin covers a group of natural chemical substances known as phosphatides. There are several kinds and modern means of processing have enabled considerable separation of individual lecithins to be achieved. They consist of various fatty acids forming phosphatidic acids with glycerophosphoric acid in esterified combination with choline, serine, inositol, or ethanolamine.

□*Natural sources* Lecithins are found throughout the animal and plant kingdoms as major cell constituents.

□*Commercial forms for supplements* Soya beans yield most of the lecithin found as granules, tablets and capsules in food supplements. Eggs are also used as a source for animal lecithins (ovolecithin) Solvent extraction processes using solvents like acetone to produce granular lecithins are sometimes criticized by the natural food enthusiasts as being too chemical.

□*Main functions* Lecithins, because of their great variety of structure, have no clearly defined role in nutrition. They are used as natural emulsifiers in foods like margarines. When broken down to smaller component parts they yield polyunsaturated fatty acids and the nutrients choline, inositol and organic phosphorus, all of which have an important role in body metabolism. As a whole they constitute nutritionally rich food elements. They are particularly recommended to aid lowering blood cholesterol levels (through their polyunsaturated fatty acids), increasing brain activity (through the choline content) and dissolving gall stones through their general emulsifying properties. Eggs contain both lecithin and cholesterol which has led some nutritionists to advocate fewer eggs to lower cholesterol, whilst others say that the beneficial effects of the lecithin far outway the danger of the cholesterol in eggs.

□*Deficiency symptoms* Lecithin in general will never be deficient, but deficiency of component elements of one or more particular lecithins may be noticed in a deficiency of choline, inositol or essential fatty acids.

□*Overdosing and toxicity* None. Reports of up to 100 g of pure lecithin daily being used nutritionally have indicated no side effects. Lecithin is a true natural food concentrate.

□*Stability* Lecithin is an oily substance, and granules may liquify and solidify as a mass if stored in a warm place.

■Octocosanol

□*Natural sources* Wheat germ.

□*Commercial sources for supplements* Octocosanol purified from wheat germ by molecular distillation, synthetic routes using long chain paraffin waxes.

□*Main functions* Stamina builder, especially in conjunction with vitamin E.

□*Deficiency symptoms* None. Octocosanol is a food factor but not a vitamin. The term pseudovitamin might be appropriate.

□*Toxicity and overdosing* None.

□*RDA* None. Supplementary quantities 2000 to 5000 mcg daily recommended by many nutritionists.

□*Co-factors* Vitamin E.

□*Stability* Very stable.

■Phosphaditinyl choline

A highly purified lecithin. Soya lecithin consists of several complex natural chemicals. Phosphaditinyl choline is obtained by special extraction and fractionation procedures from soya lecithin. In its pure form it provides a potent nutritional lecithin and a concentrated natural source of choline. It would therefore be an excellent supplement to use where additional choline is needed. (See page 90).

■RNA/DNA: Ribonucleic acid and deoxyribonucleic acid

These are the fundamental nucleic acids found in the nuclei of all living cells. DNA is the double helix compound at the root of the genetic code which controls life's processes. RNA is active in making the protein structures which actually take part in body processes. DNAs and RNAs are therefore as varied in their main structures as proteins but are only constructed from six basic interrelated compounds. These are adenine, guanine (DNA: thymine, cytosine) (RNA: uridine, cytidine). Nucleic acids also contain phosphorus and pentose sugars, as well as the basic substances mentioned. Body proteins are derived from some 22 amino acids.

□*Natural sources*   Sardines, brewer's yeast, mushrooms, green vegetables, legumes, organ meats.

□*Commercial sources for supplements*   Dried yeasts, purified animal and plant extracted nucleic acids, dried glands, dried brain.

□*Main functions*   Claims are made for the slowing of aging process, improvement of memory, particularly in older people. However, results do not convince scientists. Specific RNA/DNA injections are used by some doctors to treat aging of particular organs, but this is very controversial. It is certainly not accepted generally as a scientific treatment. All RNA-DNA is said to be digested in the stomach and only the simple components are absorbed for subsequent use in metabolism.

□*Deficiency symptoms*   RNA and DNA structures are continually built in the body and deficiency is not a possible status.

□*Co-factors*   Proteins.

□*Overdosing and toxicity*   Foods rich in these substances may cause problems to gout sufferers because breakdown of nucleic acids to purine structures may lead to high uric acid concentrations, which will exacerbate gout.

□*RDA*   None.

□*Stability*   RNA and DNA structures are stable but will largely break down in the digestive processes.

■Shell fish extracts

Oysters have long been regarded as having a beneficial effect on male potency. Inevitably oyster extracts and shells from various species have found favour in natural medicines and nutritional supplements. Oysters are rich sources of zinc, and this mineral may be their 'active' ingredient. Shell fish extracts also contain a vast number of organic substances, many of which cannot be identified.

The green-lipped mussel from New Zealand (Perna canaliculata) has recently found fame as a food supplement with beneficial effects on many forms of arthritis. Scientists are still endeavouring to discover the identity of the active ingredient. Until it is found, standardization and scientific acceptance of the extract will remain impossible. Many naturopaths and homoeopaths use the extract with success, but within an overall anti-arthritic holistic treatment programme.

Shell fish extracts carry dangers of bacterial contamination and severe allergic reactions, so be sure and choose a reliable brand and know that you are not sensitive to shell fish.

■Spirulina

Species of green algae which are harvested from unpolluted lakes generally situated high above sea level.

□*Commercial sources for supplements* Dried Mexican spirulina is said to be the best, though it is also available from other parts of the world, including Japan and Africa.

□*Main functions* As a complete vegetarian food concentrate with 65% protein and a whole spectrum of micronutrients including the B complex, betacarotene, GLA (gamma linolenic acid) and minerals. The proteins of spirulina are particularly rich in the amino acid phenylalanine, which is an appetite suppressant. Spirulina rose to fame on the story of its complete nutritional spectrum coupled with appetite suppressant properties – the ideal slimming food. The research behind it is not generally accepted and emanates only from a few doctors in the USA and Japan.

□*Deficiency symptoms* Not applicable.

□*Co-factors* Use in food supplements as a base for general vegetarian formulations is appropriate.

□*Overdosing and toxicity* None. Spirulina has been used as a food for centuries by people living in the countries where it grows.

□*RDA* None. Doses of 1 g before each meal usually recommended for people wishing to lose weight.

■Yeast

Many yeasts are found in nature. Live yeasts are used to prepare bread, wines and beers, but in consumed foods the yeast is always dead.

□*Commercial sources for supplements* Brewer's yeast, which is a by-product of brewing and is bitter in taste unless chemically treated (de-bittered). Torula yeast is cultured specially for food use and is not bitter to the taste and is generally considered nutritionally superior to brewer's yeast.

□*Main functions*   As a source of B-complex vitamins, but also proteins, nucleic acids and essential minerals.

□*Deficiency symptoms*   Not applicable.

□*Overdosing and toxicity*   Yeast is a good source of nutrients and a complete food. Some people are sensitive to yeasts and show allergic reactions. Nicotinic acid content may be sufficient to cause temporary flushing reactions in some people.

□*RDA*   None. Standardized forms of yeast are available in most countries. The contents of vitamins B1 and B2, as well as nicotinic acid, are guaranteed by adjustment of their concentrations using pure substances after analysis of the raw dried yeast; e.g. in Britain, the British Pharmacopoeia has a standard yeast which must contain the following minimum concentrations of the B vitamins:

> B1 0.1 mg/g
> B2 0.04 mg/g
> Nicotinic acid 0.3 mg/g

■10 Advertising and control of vitamins

□*Advertising and promotion*

Pick up a health food magazine in the USA and compare it with a British counterpart. You will be struck by one great difference – the informative advertising. Health problems like cancer, arthritis, sexual inadequacy are referred to, and claims to help heal sports injuries and prolong life are everywhere in the American magazine. Glowing testimonials are also liberally displayed. In the British magazine any advertisement for a vitamin or mineral supplement that tells you what it does will probably be illegal. Even claims for minor health improvements like less fatigue or fewer colds are banned. Soon we shall not even be told whether a vitamin is lost in cooking. Use of testimonials is very restricted.

The policies in the two countries represent extremes, but there must be a middle way. The present American system allows wild claims whilst the British Code of Advertising Practice leaves consumers totally puzzled and confused. Several manufacturers maintain quite large information departments to give quite simple details about their products to inviduals making personal approaches. These simple details would be illegal if presented in advertisements.

There are two basic codes of advertising practice in the UK applying to vitamins and minerals. One is controlled by the Code of Advertising Practice Committee, financed by the publishers and advertisers, and the other by the Department of Health and Social Security, who have delegated authority to various trade associations who then fund the Committee. The relevant parts of the codes are to be found on page 189.

Even in the USA pressures are being applied to prevent much of the advertising for dietary products. However, the manufacturers are a potent force with huge sales which now total over 1 billion dollars annually to finance their defence. In Britain, funds are small and the lobby against is as strong as in America. Freedoms have already been surrendered in the UK, probably to the detriment of consumers. More political pressure may well bring changes for the better.

Behind the British Advertising Committees are bureaucrats building empires with lots of sub-committees, working parties, ad hoc sub-committees, retained consultants and experts. The officials can hide behind a large smoke screen to defend a petty decision. The problem is that once these bodies are formed, only a major operation every few years, which needs to be all but fatal, will keep them in the real world.

We are not against restriction in advertising but if it is enforced without the potential advertiser being able even to talk to the decision-maker or his committee, this becomes unacceptable. In our view, the CAP Committee reached that point several years ago. Advertising has always been a political issue but it has to be accepted that in a free society a degree of freedom of information, even in the form of commercial advertising, is vitally important. The British consumer of vitamins and minerals is entitled to more informative advertising which in its turn should bring a bigger market and resources to fight the opponents of natural health food products. Many of these opponents fight from less than worthy motives. It must not be forgotten that on the CAP Committees sit doctors and experts with connections in the mainstream multinational health industries.

Most diet supplements are not subject to DHSS supervision but come under the Ministry of Agriculture, Fisheries and Foods (MAFF), because they are classed as foods not medicines. Supplements which come under the DHSS are licensed as medicines under the Medicines Act 1968. This licensing has certain commercial advantages including slightly more freedom as regards advertising and labelling. The advertisements for a licensed product will enable some deficiency claims to be made but these are not of great commercial advantage. The labelling offers greater protection. Foods have to be labelled with *all* their ingredients whilst medicines only need to have their active ingredients declared. Thus a dietary supplement capsule or tablet which has a medicines licence (PLNo) does not have to state the presence of preservatives, flavours, sugar, lactose and glycerin etc., whilst the non-licensed but identical product would have to make a full ingredient declaration, to the possible detriment of sales. So look out for the PL number statement on labels, it may assist a cover up.

With all the controls applying to dietary supplements, perhaps it is surprising the market continues to grow. However, restriction usually leads to companies trying to find ways around regulations. The health food industry has certainly spawned some ingenious schemes to achieve these ends. Some have fallen foul of the authorities, but court cases have been rare. Advertising depends so much on the interpretation of words that courts could well have impossible judgements to make.

□ *Vitamins and minerals and natural organic nutrients: the government view; regulations and codes of practice*

As you would expect in the modern world, rules and regulations surround the micronutrients just like everything else in life. As speed limits vary from country to country, so do the regulations involving micronutrients. Some governments treat vitamins and minerals in products apart from fresh food, as if they were drugs and demand controls which, whilst relevant to the novel substances which are the stock in trade of the pharmaceutical industry, have no similar meaning for natural nutrient substances. Some governments do not recognize the holistic approaches to preventive health care of the nutritional movement but look at single substance properties as regards action and toxicity quite out of context from the natural environment. We have said in the past that testing vitamins and other nutrients as if they were drugs in medical circumstances is similar to testing a bicycle for toxic exhaust fumes in the transport environment, as if it were a car. Unfortunately there are too few people who comprehend the holistic approaches to health problems to make the authorities see the futility of their policies when they insist on testing simple natural nutrients as if they were drugs.

Powerful consumer lobbies are now becoming established on behalf of the holistic natural products and it is probable that there will be greater freedom for products based on these principles in the future. Doubtless there will be a few skirmishes, but the holistic ideas are so inherently right that they just might prevail.

In the USA the vitamin industry has flourished because consumers have allied with manufacturers to force the government to relent on coercive legislation and so to favour the all powerful medical and pharmaceutical lobbies. Yet even there, constant vigilance is needed to maintain the freedom so far gained.

RDA are letters you will often see on labels of vitamins and nutrient products. They stand for *Recommended Daily Allowance*. These RDAs are drawn up by government bodies but seem to vary from country to country. Indeed we would not advise readers to take very much notice of these figures whatever country they may be in. The RDA in the USA for vitamin C is 50 to 60 mg, whilst Linus Pauling (a Nobel prize winner no less than three times – twice for chemistry) recommends over 1 gramme and himself at 80 takes some 3–5 grammes. We make no apologies for giving more credence to Pauling than to the US Government. In this book where all the nutrients are described in detail, you will find reference to RDAs where relevant, with some anomalies noted. Most items do not have RDAs because authorities do not officially recognize the essential nature of many substances.

The British Government has taken legislative action in some nutritional areas and more involvement is promised in the future. One of the oldest regulations involves the national loaf (bread). It was realized that extensive flour processing was not yielding sufficient vitamins B1, B2, B3 or the minerals calcium and iron. The Government therefore introduced regulations to ensure minimum quantities of these substances in bread loaves, and bakers added the substances at the baking stage, to ensure that the final product contained sufficient concentrations of the nutrients.

Derbyshire neck was a widespread illness which produced an underactive thyroid gland through deficiency of iodine in drinking water, particularly in parts of Derbyshire. Iodine is now added to our drinking water and this disease is no longer as common. At one time iodine was also added to table salt for the same reason, but this practice has now been discontinued. It is possible that the addition of vitamins to the national loaf may soon be discontinued too. The reasons for these changes are that people are now eating better food and no deficiencies are officially thought to exist. We disagree strongly with their reasons but agree with the action.

Fluoridation of drinking water is one of the most controversial health matters. The pro-lobby of dentists see it as a solution to British children's tooth problems and the anti-lobby are against mass medication because most people do not need to protect their teeth anyway. The fluoride that is being added in some places is sodium fluoride which is a toxic substance if taken in substantial doses. If a natural fluoride is used then things might be more acceptable.

Threats of government interference in advertising in Britain led to the setting up of the Advertising Standards Authority. This body monitors all press advertising and promotes the use of a code of practice with which all advertisements should comply (see page 189). Consumer complaints as well as official complaints on advertisements are dealt with by the authority and reports are produced regularly with firms named. As a result of complaints, advertisements have to be withdrawn and new copy submitted to the ASA before the campaign can begin again.

Advertising of medicinal products is subject to government legislation, but because of the complexity of making regulations of this kind enforceable in courts of law unless too much restriction were placed on legitimate advertisers, codes of practice are usually devised. A code operates in the nutritional field (see page 189) and this explains why so many consumers continually complain to manufacturers that they do not understand what their products are for. Whilst many manufacturers complain about this policy, it is really quite useful because it inevitably leads to people asking about nutritional products and being told that they are not like drugs but meant to be taken as part of a holistic dietary and lifestyle regime with special items being used within that regime to have particular beneficial properties.

Typical rules taken from a code of advertising practice applying to nutritional products in Britain

Submission of the proposed press advertisement to the committee shall consist of:

1 Full details of the product, including total composition, label details, leaflets and display material for use in stores.

2 Any visual matter which forms part of the advertisement as well as the full wording.

Restrictions applying to the wording

1 The immediate overall impression must be acceptable. Words which may appear misleading in headlines, even if fully interpreted in the main copy, make the advertisement unacceptable.

2 Advertisements should be factually true and supportive evidence must be supplied to the committee if requested.

3 No exaggeration, either direct or implied, is allowed.

4 No claims for cure, either direct or implied, are allowed.

5 No claims for prevention of disease except for those at special risk as given below.

  a Men and women who live alone and often do not trouble to prepare fresh or adequate meals; who tend to eat quick snacks of food which have been kept hot for long periods thus losing most of their content of some vitamins.

  b Elderly folk and others who, through various disabilities including apathy, fail to prepare or consume full varied meals.

  c Children who, because of fads, do not eat properly.

  d People who embark upon a weight reducing diet without professional advice.

  e People convalescing from an illness who have leeway to make up in their nutrition.

  f Athletes in training.

6 No offer to diagnose, advise, prescribe or treat by correspondence is allowed. (There is a widespread belief among doctors and advertising code administrators that consumers of nutritional products are likely to be hypochondriacs who are over-concerned about their health, enabling advertisers to prey on this fear.)

7 Implied content of a miraculous or mysterious, scientifically unrecognized nutritional principle is forbidden.

8 The advertisement must not discourage readers from seeking qualified medical advice. (Doctors' representatives on the advertising code committee insist on this clause.)

9 Advertisements must not appear in magazines near to editorial stories referring to the product in terms outside this code.

10 Advertisements must be clearly distinguished from editorial matter.

11 Routine, prolonged or apparent excessive use of products must be justified.

12 Responsibility for advertisements being acceptable within a code lies with both the advertiser and the publisher. They are both held equally responsible in the event of a breach of the code.

13 General health improvements related to use of the product are not allowed.

14 Confusing scientific or pseudoscientific jargon is not allowed.

15 Implication that a product is wholly or mainly natural is forbidden unless it can be shown to be derived from natural sources on that basis.

16 Claim of professional endorsement or use must be capable of just-ification but reference to doctor, dentist or pharmacist is forbidden.

17 *No advertisement shall criticize orthodox medicine or drugs.* (A good illustration of the powerful influences of those particular interests even in the nutritional field.)

18 Testimonials should be printed in full or, if abbreviated, the overall meaning must not be altered. Testimonials over three years old may not be used in press or TV advertisements but seven-year-old ones are permitted in leaflets and catalogues not included in product packs.

19 Testimonials containing claims disallowed by any part of the overall code are forbidden.

Restrictions applying to illustrations and graphs

1 No graph which could be interpreted in terms leading to con-travention of forbidden written copy is allowed.

2 Pictures of doctors, nurses, dentists, pharmacists or other health professionals are forbidden.

Restrictions applied to books sold in conjunction with nutritional supplements

If a book is offered for sale or is even mentioned within a product advertisement, then the title and any reference to contents must not amount to a product claim forbidden by the code.

Persons to whom this code applies

It must be remembered that so far as health is concerned the only professional bodies recognized are doctors, dentists and pharmacists. Other groups can be informed through advertising of only a relatively restricted area of medicine. This code will therefore apply to advertisements directed at all groups who are not recognized as qualified practitioners, e.g. chiropractors, naturopaths, osteopaths, physiotherapists, chiropodists, opticians, dietitians, nutritionists, health store proprietors, and others.

□ *The Code of Advertising Practice (UK)*
usually referred to as CAP Code

This booklet is regularly updated and includes sections embracing every facet of press advertising (newspapers and magazines). Another code, in many ways similar to the CAP code, applies to TV and radio. Copies of the codes are available from the relevant bodies (see Appendix).

On health matters both practice committees rely heavily on medical experts. It is hardly surprising that we find the views of the medical establishment dominating the resulting codes and deliberations for pre-vetting of advertisements.

These particularly apposite extracts, taken from Appendix K of the Code, illustrate the dominance of the official and medical view and speak for themselves.

1.1 Vitamins and minerals are essential at all ages for the maintenance of physical and mental health and well-being. The daily requirements for normal healthy individuals are available from a full, properly varied and well-prepared diet. It is unnecessary therefore for such a diet to be supplemented by the taking of extra vitamins or minerals, and it is unlikely that there would be any benefit from so

189

doing. Too much of certain vitamins, e.g. vitamin D, and some minerals can be harmful. Vitamin deficiencies, however, can occur but they are mostly multiple and deficiencies of single vitamins are less usual. Iron deficiency can occur among women of child-bearing age who may need more than is provided by their normal diet.

1.2 In cases of serious illness, e.g. following surgical operation and in certain diseases, an individual's intake or utilization of dietary vitamins and minerals may be impaired and the intake needs to be augmented. The prescriptions of vitamins and minerals in those cases should be the province of the doctor, and self-medication should not be encouraged.

1.4 In assessing the adequacy of the formulation of vitamin and mineral products, the Committee will have regard to the recommended daily intakes published by the DHSS.

> Thiamin *1.1 mg*
> Riboflavin *1.7 mg*
> Nicotinic acid (Niacin) *18 mg*
> Ascorbic acid *30 mg*
> Vitamin A, *750 mcg (2,500 iu)*
> Vitamin D *2.5 mcg (100 iu)*
> Iron *10 mg*

Advertisement claims

4.1 Cases of serious vitamin/mineral deficiency can be recognized only on medical examination and may require treatment by therapeutic dosages prescribed for the individual's needs, and self-medication should not be encouraged.

Unacceptable claims

4.2 The following are examples of claims and implications regarding the value of the vitamin/mineral content of products, which are undesirable in advertisements addressed to the public:

> **1** That a full, varied and properly prepared diet needs to be supplemented with extra vitamins or minerals.
> **2** That the taking of products providing extra vitamins/minerals will benefit everybody.
> **3** That there is evidence of general, widespread vitamin/mineral deficiency.
> **4** That good looks and good health can be maintained or achieved only by taking extra vitamins or minerals.

5 That irritability, nerviness and lack of energy are caused only by vitamin-mineral deficiencies.
6 That the taking of extra vitamins or minerals hastens recovery from infections such as colds and influenza, or that it will protect the individual from contracting such ailments.

■11 Micronutrients in commerce

As knowledge of the precise nature of nutrients has evolved, so has their use in consumer products and medicines.

It is now a regular occurrence for foods to be labelled 'with added vitamins and minerals'. A vitamins-added claim is useful copy for successful advertisements for food products on TV and in magazines. Whatever the opinions of the national bodies who tell us how balanced and adequate in nutrients is the diet they advocate for us and which we are all supposed to be eating, it seems that many consumers feel that it is worth paying extra for 'added vitamins'.

Breakfast cereals are probably the most conspicuous product area for the addition of vitamins, but micronutrient fortified flours and milks are used in the food industry to produce a host of specialist foods for slimmers, sportsmen, body builders and the health-aerobics oriented people. These foods are becoming more and more important sources of revenue and are moving from specialist stores to the supermarket and chains. Specialist magazines on health, slimming, diet and exercise are increasing. Established publications often produce regular features and may even produce occasional supplements to see whether their market is ready for a full blown new health magazine.

Let us look at the main areas in more detail.

□Slimming products

There are two main kinds, the meal replacers and the appetite satisfiers. The meal replacers are those temptingly labelled 'X Day Diet Plans' or sachet packed snacks with less calories. Every year seems to bring a new platform for the advertisers, but the powders remain very much the same: milk protein concentrates artificially sweetened and with added vitamins and minerals to meet official recommended daily allowances. Instructions are changed and perhaps the new 'special ingredient' is added or a new dietary description is used. Most readers will recall the Scarsdale diet, the grapefruit diet, the Beverley Hills diet etc. All depend on one basic fact, the reduction of calories to below 1000 a day.

The appetite satisfier will be a bulking agent such as a cellulose, gum, pectin or cereal fibre. These may be presented as capsules, tablets or sachets. When taken with water they fill the stomach and prevent you eating calories. They are a crutch to that vital thing, keeping below 1000 calories a day. Often they are boosted with micronutrients to ensure that you get the recommended daily allowances despite only taking 1000 calories worth of food.

Slimming clubs and magazines help you because they assure you that there are others out there with the same aims. You can share your experience with them, which is a very important social need in itself.

There are only two ways to lose weight, eating less or exercising more. Both methods reduce stored calories in whatever form, fat, carbohydrate or protein, because all are interchangeable.

Water loss to lose weight is different and can be achieved easily with mild natural diuretics like dandelion, boldo and seaweed extracts. It is not strictly a 'nutritional way to lose weight', it is a medical treatment and needs care. Many women suffer from bloating during particular points in the menstrual cycle and by careful dietary adjustment can minimize this problem. One method is to decrease salt intake and increase potassium. There are many treatments and supplements on the market too.

□ *Complementary medicine products*

The term 'complementary' or 'alternative' has been widely adopted to apply generally to forms of medical treatment that are largely outside the kind usually available on the National Health Service. Homoeopathy is the only branch of complementary medicine which is available in some areas on the National Health Service.

Osteopathy, herbal medicine, chiropractic and acupuncture are the better-known complementary medicine methods.

Nutritional therapies usually form an integral part of complementary treatments but the addition of vitamins and minerals is not universal. There are general dietary recommendations to cut out red meat, increase fibre, reduce saturated fat, cut down salt, cut out processed foods, watch for synthetic food additives, cut refined sugar and white flour. These are the usual approaches. Few practitioners in the complementary field stray into the areas of vitamin therapy because, as professionals, they fear that their knowledge is not sufficient in that area. They would probably all prefer supplementary vitamins to drugs because they understand that vitamins and minerals are substances which the body understands, any side effects being likely to be transitory and reversible. Such confidence in drugs is impossible.

Many complementary practitioners are now learning about the help that vitamins and minerals can give their patients and are taking courses from both American and British institutions. We can expect considerable growth of interest from these professionals in the future.

Some manufacturers of herbal and homoeopathic medicines have added vitamins and minerals to their formulas. The rationales behind these products are usually little more than marketing ploys. The concept of biochemical individuality which pervades most complementary medical practice, demands specific supplements or homoeopathic and herbal products for each individual. There are no truly general treatment products of this kind.

□ *Official medicinal uses for vitamins and minerals*

Diseases such as beriberi and rickets will be treated with the appropriate vitamins because there is scientific proof of their being vitamin-deficiency diseases. Equally, pernicious anaemia will be treated with vitamin B12 injections. Complete control or cures will be obtained without side effects. If a drug treatment directly interferes with vitamin availability (see Folic acid, page 86) then supplements are an appropriate additional item of treatment. Prescription of vitamins or minerals for other purposes is comparatively rare. Indeed, medical authorities with socialized schemes such as the UK Department of Health and Social Security restrict ad lib prescribing of vitamins and tonics. They take the view that the balanced diet provides enough vitamins. Supplements providing what they consider enough for the 'at risk groups' (see page 187) are very low dose synthetics. In the right circumstances they will permit official prescribing of such products. The naturally-based products with higher concentrations of scheduled vitamins and minerals together with a whole spectrum of non-approved and pseudonutrients are not allowed.

A doctor who prescribes vitamins outside the approved range often has to justify his actions to a committee. If they are not satisfied, they will penalize him. A doctor in the British National Health Service can prescribe anything, even whisky, but if the product falls outside the approved list and the doctor fails to justify its use, he or she can be in serious trouble. Clinical freedom is a closely guarded privilege amongst doctors. It is a very hot political potato in these days of socialized medicine because clever marketing by commercial interests can exploit this 'freedom' to the detriment of tax-payers. Vitamin and mineral supplements is one of the areas where, understandably, authorities have thought it important to intervene.

□*Proprietary vitamins and tonics*

These products form the major part of the market in vitamins and minerals. The natural supplements are sold mainly in health food stores and the synthetic ones sold in chemists, drug stores and supermarkets. This division is blurred and, as has been shown in the individual sections on nutrients themselves, synthetic methods of production permeate all areas. However, most natural vitamin manufacturers try to make products more closely approaching a natural food whilst those offering the wholly synthetic products prepare them as if they were drugs.

The major brands currently advertised on television are mainly synthetic in content and concept. They are cheaper to produce and so more money can be expended on their promotion. In newspapers and magazines, the natural vitamin will be advertised, but strict rules surrounding the wording of all promotional material including leaflets make appreciation of the benefits of the naturally conceived product difficult to get across to consumers. This means that market growth tends to be enjoyed by the synthetic brands and these are usually totally out of line with good natural dietary ideals. They often contain sugar, synthetic colours, flavours, preservatives, plasticizers, binders, emulsifiers and some are even made effervescent by use of a host of chemical agents. Children's vitamins are often the worst in these respects. This is alarming because many people believe additives are a contributory factor to hyperactivity and mental disturbances in the young.

The major synthetic brands tend to be fairly low in strength and this has led to unfair comparison of prices between health stores and chemists. Journalists pick up a weak multivitamin from a chemist and compare its price with a stronger natural multivitamin in the health food store. They then infer, quite unfairly, that the health store is ripping the consumer off. Would they go to a car showroom of a mass brand dealer and to a Rolls Royce dealer and make a similar statement, simply on the basis that both products had four wheels and an engine? If this book has achieved anything, then it will have educated people about the real and apparent differences between vitamin supplement products.

Many tonics are liquid products, but again the synthetic brands will be different from the natural ones. A careful reading of the labels will tell you which is which: the medicine will have its Product Licence No. and a little information, whilst the natural product will have a full list of predominantly wholesome ingredients.

□*Special diet foods*

There are many meal replacers and special foods on the market for people on restricted diets for reasons of illness or infirmity. However, sometimes their nutritional composition leaves much to be desired.

The use of breast-milk substitutes is declining in many developed countries because mothers have come to realize that 'Breast is Best'. There is no real substitute for breast milk because this not only gives nutrition but also passes immunity to many diseases from mother to baby. Neither cow's milk, goat's or soya can do both these things. Manufacture of breast milk substitutes is big business and producers try to keep their brands up to date with current nutritional research. Vitamins and minerals as well as amino acid profiles are very important. We have already made a comparison of the nutritional profile of mother's milk and a leading substitute and it well illustrates the problems confronting manufacturers trying to make a satisfactory product (page 39).

Don't forget that our knowledge of nutrition is growing all the time and what may be a substance or balance of substances which appears of little consequence today can assume a major baby health role tomorrow.

Special gluten-free dietary products are manufactured to cater for coeliac disease sufferers. This is an illness where malabsorption of food takes place because of sensitivity to the protein fraction in wheat known as gluten/gliadin. This is also found in rye, barley and oats. Sufferers have to avoid all cereal and baked products likely to contain gluten/gliadin, which includes bread and cakes. Many of the special foods are made from an industrial by-product wheat starch from which practically all the gluten/gliadin has been removed. When the gluten-gliadin is being removed, all the other nutrients (vitamins and minerals) which are rich in wholewheat go too. When manufacturers make their flours and special breads, it seems that not enough effort is made to put back all the micronutrients lost in the processing. So the coeliac patient has a staple food denuded of nearly all its nutrients yet containing traces of his toxin gluten/gliadin. (By coincidence, the same product is used for starching clothes in laundries.) Why this is allowed to happen when wholefood substitutes for wheat flour are readily available remains a mystery but less than worthy motives may well lie behind it all.

Problems arise with low protein foods but again the progress in nutritional knowledge gives the manufacturers little chance to keep their products up to date. So if you are on a special diet, be sure to look at the foods prescribed and take precautions to top up likely deficiencies of micronutrients with supplements or find wholefoods which meet your dietary requirements.

□*Body-building products*

By this term we mean the foods which are used as concentrates by muscle builders and athletes. Body-builders need to have a highly specialized diet to achieve the muscle structure and definition they require. They expend a great deal of energy in the exercise regimes necessary for the achievement of their goals. So the diet must provide for both rapid energy release and structural growth.

Basic diets rich in high protein foods such as meat, eggs and liver are followed, but it is the all important supplements which can give competitors the edge in performance. Commercially, these consist of powders for incorporating in milk or water, canned protein drinks and the familiar tablets, capsules and sachets of individual or multiple micronutrients as concentrates.

Body-building magazines are proliferating on bookstalls and articles promote a great variety of diet and exercise regimes which have been adopted by the successful muscle builders of both sexes. In America, diets in this area are almost as numerous as in the slimming field. It all points to bio-chemical individuality again. It is really no use going from diet to diet but better to take a good basic one and adapt it to your own particular needs. Not easy, but then was success at anything ever simple? The vitamin and mineral products promoted specially for body-builders and athletes are often the same as the general brands but with a different label and probably at a higher price. High strength vitamin and mineral capsules and tablets are openly promoted to the body-building fraternity, but the extra expense of the extra potency will not usually be justified in practice.

Quality protein foods are vitally important to the body-builder. The canned liquid protein is a very expensive product but the powders are much more economical. Milk and egg powders are used with various balances promoted commercially as more desirable than others. As more is learned about individual amino acids which are the building blocks of all proteins, a scientific basis for different basic protein mixtures may be found. At present only individual results will dictate the use of a particular brand.

Provided a powder contains more than 50% protein, then we would consider the best buy would be the one which gave you the most weight of protein for your money. It would be better to buy 500 g of 60% protein than 300 g of 90% for the same price. After all, the 500 g would be giving you 40% of other nutrients too which could well be the instant energy sources (carbohydrate-glucose) you need for daily training sessions.

Amino acids are receiving more attention from nutritionists and doctors. Commercially the pure amino acids are developing substantial markets and in no area is their potential more readily exploited than body-building. There is great scope for pseudoscience but perhaps some of the ideas may not be far wide of the mark. Growth hormone release by arginine/ornithine is one interesting aspect. The amino acids are taken in large doses on their own to activate the body's own muscle growth stimulators. It is possible that particular protein balances established by trial and error in body-building diets have provided particular amino acid balances after digestion which have activated body-building metabolic processes rather than just provided the building blocks – i.e., perhaps they provide the bricklayers as well as the bricks!

□*Processed foods*

Ironically the processing of foods which depletes wholesome starting materials of much of their nutritional value as far as micronutrients are concerned, provides a commercial outlet for vitamins and minerals involving many thousands of tons annually. The expression 'with added vitamins' is surprising on breakfast cereals prepared from a starting material which has been de-husked. Even fibre is added back to some products. The trouble is that even after the adding back, nutritional balance is not restored because the 'whole' spectrum of nutrients is not put back, only those which are recognized as essential by the authorities. They work several years behind research results and represent not only government but vested commercial processing interests.

A good example of processing is white flour from whole wheat. Table 1 shows what happens during processing. Commercial bread made from white flour is currently fortified to restore just the B1, niacin and iron contents. Calcium is added too, but to a greater extent than it was in the whole wheat. This is because there was a widespread view at one time that calcium deficiency was caused by the ingestion of too much bread. Wheat contains phytic acid which is a chemical binder of calcium and is said to prevent its absorption. Recent research has cast doubt on this proposition, so it may no longer be necessary to add calcium to bread flour.

Illustration of approximate losses and gains in nutrients in processing of a food – wholewheat flour – into white flour in mg per 100 g unless stated otherwise:

nutrient	wholewheat flour	white processed flour	difference	% difference
protein g	13.2	9.8	−3.4	−26
potassium mg	360	140	−120	−33
calcium mg*	35	150	+115	+330
magnesium mg	140	20	−120	−86
phosphorus mg	340	110	−230	−68
iron mg*	4	2.4	−1.6	−40
copper mg	0.4	0.2	−0.2	−50
zinc mg	3.0	0.7	−2.3	−77
vitamin B6 mg	0.5	0.2	−0.3	−66
folic acid mcg	57	22	−35	−60
pantothenic acid mg	0.8	0.3	−0.5	−63
biotin mcg	7	1	−6	−86
vitamin B1 mg*	0.46	0.33	−0.13	−28
vitamin B2 mg	0.08	0.02	−0.06	−75
vitamin B3 mg*	5.6	2.0	−3.6	−64
vitamin E mg	1.0	*trace*	*approx* −1.0	−95 (at least)
fibre g	9.6	3.4	−6.2	−65

These items are boosted by law after milling (UK), so some losses are made good. See page 198 regarding why there is more calcium in processed than unprocessed wheat flour.

Additives in processed foods may also deprive the food of micronutrients, but equally they may prolong the life of others. In either case balance is disturbed, but whether this is harmful remains doubtful.

■12 Conclusions and the future

'A growing market with 'products in tune with the trendy philosophy put across by the "Green" political movement.'

Perhaps such a phrase could apply to the health food and nutritional supplement industry as it is in 1985. Natural nutrient products are seen as good by many people, but if we are not careful they will be given a reputation which may prove very fragile.

Many companies use expressions such as 'natural', 'not tested on animals', 'preservative free', 'additive free', 'organically grown', without being sure. These statements could be challenged with success in probably more than 90% of instances. In America some of the claims regarding purity and naturalness are already ridiculous. An American product containing pollen was described as having all its ingredients coming from unpolluted areas – an impossible guarantee unless you traced every member of the hive on its tour collecting pollen. You would also have to check the people sent to do the collection of the pollen. The French use 'appellation controlée' to try and enforce wine standards. Nothing resembling this surrounds any raw material used in health foods or supplements apart from ginseng where the Koreans have tried a scheme with mixed results.

Consumers must be vigilant and ask manufacturers to justify claims. One letter of a technical nature will sort out the genuine producer. If you either do not get a reply or just a woolly answer, then they will have told you enough to make up your own mind.

The expression 'not tested on animals' is very misleading. Whilst the company itself may not have tested the ingredients used in its products on animals, if it is a government approved food or cosmetic ingredient, then at some time it will have been tested on animals. It would be illegal to use non-approved ingredients in most countries. Just because a particular manufacturer or seller has not done a test is meaningless and misleading. Indeed of all the expressions used in marketing natural products, this must be one that is always wrong.

If any reader can dispute this statement with factual data, the authors will look forward to hearing from them.

The natural food movement may be going forward, but industry inevitably needs to foster growth. Accountants make calculations of growth to impress shareholders and financiers. They cannot rely upon the unknown. Commercial methods based upon the science of economics should be brought into the picture so that a guaranteed minimum growth can be achieved. The fact that their scientifically based predictions are hardly ever fulfilled does not stop accountants and economists. They ask the marketing departments to ensure their budgeted sales increase takes place. In many industries this can be achieved because marketing strategies are not surrounded with too many regulations and patents operate. However, in the natural nutrients area, huge constraints operate in the vital advertising and promotional field (see page 187) and the only form of patent is a trade mark. How the industry is reacting to these circumstances is quite intriguing.

Let us look at the areas of trademark exploitation. A mark can be applied to a single product or to a large group. If one takes a single product mark it can only be developed by use of informative advertising and promotion. In the health food industry informative advertising and promotion is impossible, so this method is a non-starter. Using group marks, the only thing one can sell is superior quality and service – an angle which may increase your sales within the total but is unlikely to expand the overall market. But it is expansion of the overall market which is needed, so we come back to the single product mark as the only real solution.

In the last ten years, there have been some real successes in the nutritional concentrate field. How were these successes achieved in the face of the regulations? It is safe to say that none was achieved within the strict rules. The technique used by the companies was to promote their trade mark in close proximity to the accepted generic title. They also tried to ensure that most of the raw material initially available was supplied exclusively to them at a very competitive price.

Whilst the policy succeeded in the short term when they were spending a great deal of money on press releases and conferences as well as radio and TV interviews, in the medium term trouble lay ahead. New sources of raw material became available and generic producers who had spent nothing on promotion took the all important growth slice of the market in that product. Thanks to the efforts of the innovating companies the market has grown, but how many in the future are going to take the same risks with no long-term reward?

The use of books and magazines to publicize nutrients is well established in both America and Britain. Perhaps this is not a very good thing but it is inevitable in an industry surrounded by hostile regulatory authorities. Freedom of the written and spoken word is a vital part of our way of life. People feel strongly that natural nutrients can help health problems but they know that proof to satisfy the authorities and doctors, whilst obtainable, would not be economically viable because no patent protection could be provided. This means that there is no ultimate return on an original investment – a very difficult point for most people to understand. The makers use the freedom provided in the publishing area to ensure that information which may be scientifically unacceptable reaches the public. They feel that their actions are fully justified whilst the medical establishment and its friends in the multinational pharmaceutical industry have failed to achieve their promise of universal health for all. Indeed, many feel that those promised cures are getting further away and that the side effects of the treatments and products could be getting out of hand in some areas.

The risks the health food manufacturers take are great because if their opponents found a single fault in their products and ideas, serious problems could arise. Already it is quite evident that as soon as there is a favourable article about vitamins in the press, it is not long before the other view is put. We have seen it even with major food products such as sugar and salt where, as soon as one group is saying reduce, there are others saying there is no harm in the amounts already being consumed.

Progress for the natural food and nutrient industry has been steady and we are sure that it will continue, provided nobody is tempted by any more short term wonder substances like DMSO (see page 173). If all products marketed are genuine nutrients, then positive contribution to health in the future will be made.

■Appendix

Technical terms and useful information

■Technical Terms

Although we have taken great pains to present the information in this book in a very simple way, some jargon has had to be used. Here is a list to help you understand just what the jargon means.

Transit time – the length of time it takes for food to pass right through the body.

Alimentary canal – the digestive tract (the food tube).

EFA – Essential Fatty Acids, also known as polyunsaturates.

Atherosclerosis – hardening of the arteries.

NACNE – National Advisory Committee for Nutrition Education.

Organic – any chemical substance based upon the carbon atom.

Thrombosis – formation of blood clots.

Orotate – the orotic acid form of a mineral.

RDA – Recommended Daily Allowance/Amount, usually backed by government authority.

g – gramme (1/1000 part of a kilo); 28 g = 1 oz approx.

mg – milligramme (1/1000 part of a gramme).

mcg – microgramme (1/1000 part of a milligramme), also denoted as μg.

iu – international unit, a measure of quantity applied to vitamins, but it does not equal the same weight for all vitamins.

Krebs Cycle – the metabolic process the body uses to convert glucose to energy.

Electrolyte – a chemical substance which conducts electricity. Its components are positively and negatively charged.

Neuritis – inflammation of nerves.

Anorexia – disease that causes people to stop eating or slowly starve by eating an insufficient amount of food. Associated with young girls who take slimming too seriously and carry dieting to extremes.

Oxidative processes – metabolic processes involving oxygen.

Lactation – breast feeding.

Vasodilator – natural enlarger of blood vessels.

Corticosteroid hormones – hormones produced in the cortex of the adrenal gland.

Immune system – the body's defence system.

Mucosa – cells on surface of organs such as the mouth, stomach, intestines, lungs.

D or L – these capital letters immediately before a chemical name indicate whether it is dextro (right-handed) or laevo (left-handed) in form and refers to the direction in which its molecules bend polarized light. In nature, the L forms seem to predominate for amino acids, whilst the D forms predominate for vitamins.

Microflora – the friendly bacteria found in the human intestine, usually lactobacilli.

Hygroscopic – picks up moisture on exposure to air.

Halogen – the group of elements comprising fluorine, bromine, chlorine and iodine.

Sulpha drug – the group of antibacterial drugs based on the sulphonamide structure.

Crustacea – crabs, lobsters, prawns, scampi, shrimps.

Molluscs – shellfish, snails, mussels, oysters, cockles.

Pathogenic bacteria – bacteria which cause disease.

Micronutrients – vitamins, minerals and trace elements found in foods.

pH – a measure of the acidity or alkalinity of a solution. Less than 7 is acid, more than 7 is alkaline.

Esterified – the combination of an organic alcohol with an organic acid.

GDU – General Digestive Units.

MFU – McCord and Fridovitch Units.

■Calcium and Osteoporosis

Due to the menopause the levels of oestrogen fall in a woman's body. This results in a gradual loss of calcium from the bones in the years following the menopause. As the bones become more brittle they tend to fracture more easily than in younger women. Supplementing the diet of women over the age of 45 with calcium can help to combat the problem. Magnesium and Vitamin D are also needed to help with the calcium absorption.

■Useful information

■Further reading

Tables in this book are based on information from *The Composition of Foods*, Medical Research Council (HMSO, 4th edition, 1978).

Other useful books are:

Manual of Nutrition, The Ministry of Agriculture, Fisheries and Food (HMSO, 8th edition, 1976).

Don't Forget Fibre in the Diet, Denis Burkitt (M. Dunitz, 4th edition, 1983).

The British Food Fiasco, Rita Greer (Bunterbird Ltd, 1984).

The Right Way to Cook, Rita Greer (Dent, 1985).

■Useful addresses

Advertising Standards Authority
3 Brook House
Torrington Place
London WC1E 7HN

Independent Broadcasting Authority
70 Brompton Road
London SW3 1EY

■Index

A
acerola 63
acid
  arachidonic 29
  essential fatty (EFAs) 29, 102
  gamma linolenic 29, 102
  lauric 29
  linoleic 29, 102
  linolenic 29
  myristic 29
  oleic 29
  palmitic 29
  stearic 29
acidophilus 167
additives
  in food 53
  in supplements 61–65
adenine (B4) 76–77
advertising 183
  code of practice 189
  standards authority 186
alanine 140–141
alcohol 146, 158
alfalfa 165
allergies 55
aloe vera 167–168
aluminium 136
amino acids 11, 36, 37, 52, 55,
    139–163
  alanine 140–141
  arginine 141–142
  aspartic acid 143
  citrulline 144
  cysteine 145–146
  cystine 144–145
  DL-Phenylalanine 154–155
  GABA, Gamma amino
    butyric acid 146
  glutamine and glutamic
    acid 146–147
  glycine 147–148
  histidine 148–149
  isoleucine 149
  L-Phenylalanine 154–155
  L-tyrosine 161–162
  leucine 150
  lysine 151
  methionine 152–153
  ornithine 154

  proline 156–157
  serine 157–158
  taurine 158
  threonine 158–159
  tryptophan 159–161
  valine 162–163
amygdalin (B17) 84–85
amylase 165
anaemia 8, 85, 116
aneurine (B1) 71
arginine 141–142
arsenic 137
ascorbic acid 92–96
aspartic acid 143–144

B
bacteria, helpful 11
barium 136
bee products 168–170
beta carotene 57
betaine 170
bicarbonates 171
bile 11
  salts 11, 158
bilious attack 13
biocytin 103–105
bioflavoniod 64, 105–106
biotin (Vit H) 103–105
boldo 52
boron 108
brans
  oat 16
  pea 16
  rice 16
  seed 16
  soya 16
  wheat 16, 20
bread 43, 186
  recipe 44
breast milk 38–39
bromelain 166
bromine 108

C
cadmium 51
calcium 54, 64, 109–111, 198
  and osteoporosis *see*
    Appendix
CAP committee 184